Mutual care in

Palliative
MEDICINE

A STORY OF DOCTORS AND PATIENTS

Dedicated to those people whose stories form the basis of this book, and to my family

Platon Vafiadis

Mutual care in

Palliative
MEDICINE

A STORY OF DOCTORS AND PATIENTS

McGRAW-HILL BOOK COMPANY Sydney

New York San Francisco Auckland Bogotá Caracas
Lisbon London Madrid Mexico City Milan Montreal
New Delhi San Juan Singapore Tokyo Toronto

McGraw·Hill Australia

A Division of The McGraw·Hill Companies

National Library of Australia Cataloguing-in-Publication data:

Vafiadis, Platon.
Mutual care in palliative medicine: a story of doctors and patients.

Bibliography.
ISBN 0 074 71066 4.

1   Palliative treatment. 2. Physician and patient.
I   Title.

362.175

Published in Australia by
McGraw-Hill Book Company Australia Pty Limited
4 Barcoo Street, Roseville NSW 2069, Australia
Publishing Manager: Meiling Voon
Production Editor: Sybil Kesteven
Editor: Frith Luton
Interior and Cover Design: Jenny Pace Design
Illustrator: Alan Laver, Shelly Communications
Cover image: Digital Vision
Typeset in Bembo by Jenny Pace Design
Printed on 80gsm woodfree by Prowell Productions, Hong Kong.

Contents

LIST OF FIGURES, TABLES AND BOXES   vii
PREFACE   ix

Introduction   1

The social history of medical power and the doctor–patient relationship   2
The return of power to the patient: behaviour in health and illness   4
Models of the doctor–patient relationship   6
Medical power and the delivery of medical care   8
The compatibility of medical power with doctor–patient equality:
    current challenges   10
The 'new' doctor   11
The 'new' patient   14
Statement of the problem   15
A framework for examining issues of authority in the
    doctor–patient relationship   18
Implementation of the research framework   20
Conclusion: towards the cancer experience   20

Chapter 1

Illness Through the Eyes of Patient and Doctor   21
The cancer world of patient and carer   22
The cancer world of the clinician   46
Conclusion: towards unifying patient and doctor experiences   61

Chapter 2

Doctor–Family Interaction   63
The pre-consultation period   65
The medical diagnostic process   66
The nature and purpose of disclosure   69
Awareness in disclosure   69
Dynamics of disclosure   72
Emotive and non-verbal content of disclosure   75
Should disclosure focus primarily on knowledge or on coping?   75
Treatment as 'active' or 'passive'   76
The 'activity' of non-medical forms of treatment   80
Synchronising the notions of 'activity' and 'passivity' in treatment   81
Monitoring of progress   82

Adjustment to transition   85
Site of care: the home versus the hospital   87
Interaction, change and uncertainty: summary and implications for
    medical power   90
Prerequisites for doctor–patient harmony: an insight into the nature
    of medical power   93
Conclusion: the effects of uncertainty on doctor–patient compatibility   96

Chapter 3

The Challenge of Medical Uncertainty   98
Knowledge-related uncertainty   99
Implications of knowledge-related uncertainty   102
Uncertainty related to health-care structure   103
Implications of uncertainty related to health-care structure   105
Process-related uncertainty   105
Implications of process-related uncertainty   113
Inherent medical uncertainty   113
Implications of inherent medical uncertainty   116
Uncertainty in the negotiation of different paradigms of illness   116
Implications of uncertainty in the negotiation of different paradigms of illness 117
Moral and emotional uncertainty   118
Implications of moral and emotional uncertainty   120
Uncertainty in the clinical context: an overview   121
Conclusion: the concept of doctor–patient distance   124

Chapter 4

Distance, Ownership and Role Reversal in Clinical Relationships   126
Interpersonal distance between doctor and patient   127
Professional distance   127
Social distance   132
Emotional distance   135
Refining the concept of distance: the notion of ownership   137
Role reversal: an introduction   144
Role reversal: a description   146
Role reversal: a summary and comparative analysis   149
Distance, ownership and role reversal, and implications for medical power 154
Conclusion: towards a new model of the clinical encounter   157

Chapter 5

**Bi-Directional Care Between Doctor and Patient:
A New Model**   159
The nature and quality of medical power: a summary   159
Bi-Directional Care: a model of GP–patient interaction in palliative care 167
Conclusion: the significance of mutual care   176

CONCLUSION   178
APPENDIX   182
BIBLIOGRAPHY   186
INDEX   193

List of figures, tables and boxes

Box I.1 Key elements of the Health Belief Model   4
Box I.2 Key elements of the Model of Illness Behaviour   5
Box I.3 Ajzen's Theory of Planned Behaviour   5
Box I.4 Doctor and patient roles   6
Box I.5 A model of the doctor–patient relationship according to level
of control   7
Box I.6 A model of the doctor–patient relationship according to level of
participation   7
Box I.7 Enhancing and utilising cultural awareness in clinical practice   9
Box I.8 The patient-centred method   9
Box 1.1 Patient and carer emphases on cancer   22
Box 1.2 Emphasis placed on cancer by GPs   47
Table 1.1 Time-orientations of different palliative care approaches   53
Table 1.2 *Functional* versus **epidemiological** modes of medical response   53
Box 2.1 Sequences of illness progression   64
Box 2.2 Awareness contexts in terminal illness   70
Figure 2.1 Possible directions in disclosure   72
Box 2.3 Key prerequisites for doctor–patient harmony   94
Box 3.1 Major categories of medical uncertainty   99
Figure 3.1 Models for diagnostic delay   109
Box 4.1 Key issues linking distance to ownership   138
Box 4.2 Doctor-patient ownership and distance according to socially
prescribed roles   144
Figure 4.1 Direction of care   145
Box 4.3 Key features of role reversal   149
Box 5.1 Key unanswered issues in medical power   159
Figure 5.1 The patient-centred clinical method   167
Figure 5.2 Bi-Directional Care: foundations   168
Figure 5.3 Bi-Directional Care: effects of continuity   170
Figure 5.4 The Model of Bi-Directional Care   173
Figure 5.5 Links between doctor–patient distance and role reversal over time 173
Table A.1 Summary of family informants   184
Table A.2 Summary of General Practitioner informants   185
Table A.3 Informants who completed formal interviews   185

Preface

Modern medicine has grown remarkably in the last half-century. Progressive advances in pharmacology, immunology, pathophysiology and diagnostic and imaging technology have made possible feats that would have been inconceivable only a short while ago. Within the span of a single lifetime, the appearance of antibiotics and vaccines has bolstered earlier advances in nutrition and hygiene to alter dramatically the impact of infectious diseases in the developed world. Within fifty years after the discovery of deoxyribonucleic acid (DNA), genetic engineering and gene therapy are now well established pursuits within molecular biology. Changes in surgical technique have also been as revolutionary, exemplified through minimally invasive 'keyhole' surgery, advances in intricate microsurgical reconstructive techniques, surgery on the unborn child, and multiple organ transplantation. The public imagination has been captured by the seemingly invincible potential of medicine to advance and to cure.

Medicine, however, has paid a price for this rather glamorous image. It has engendered expectations that it struggles to live up to, since it cannot cure many forms of disease. Advancing technology has also outpaced moral debate, generating ethical dilemmas across all sub-disciplines of medicine. Issues such as in-vitro fertilisation and embryo experimentation and storage, the initial access and then the criteria for turning off life-support machines, the emotional and ethical consequences of genetic screening, the implications of false positive and false negative test results, or even the potential stigma associated with a 'positive' test result are all weighty issues which threaten to de-humanise medical practice. Quite apart from these issues, the increasing complexity of medicine carries implications for the extent to which patient consent is truly informed. Increasing sophistication and complexity have also generated huge increases in health-care costs and added additional time pressures to an already time-starved discipline. Furthermore, new drugs and procedures often carry higher risks of mortality and morbidity to coincide with their increased potential to improve health. It is little wonder, then, that chinks have started to appear in the seemingly impregnable armour of medicine.

A major question is naturally generated from this state of affairs: How is medicine able to reconcile its advanced knowledge and expertise with its very real limitations and shortcomings? This work pursues this question by specifically examining medical authority (or power) as it is manifested and lived in the doctor–patient relationship. It is at the personal level, at the face-to-face interaction between doctor and patient, where the emotional tension of reconciling expertise with limitation is felt most strongly. Unlike a failed laboratory experiment, which is impersonal and can therefore be safely relegated to the past without any emotional cost, failure at the person-to-person level carries emotional repercussions that may be impossible to reverse.

As a general practitioner I have often experienced the fragility of medical authority first-hand. I wrote this book because I found that many clinical situations present complex challenges that cannot be addressed by the patient-centred approach, even though the latter is a 'gold-standard' model taught to health professionals the world over.

Important questions about medical authority at the individual level have several facets. What form does medical authority or power take? How does the medical profession deal with failure, uncertainty, adverse side effects or the inability to cure? What impact do these points have upon patients and doctors, upon their perception of the medical process, and upon the nature and stability of their association? These issues hold the key to a better understanding of the doctor–patient relationship, including the innermost intricacies of its dynamics, and ultimately the nature of medical practice itself. This work examines these issues in six sections.

The Introduction overviews the social history and evolution of medical power with specific reference to how it has influenced the doctor–patient relationship. It then highlights current limitations in the understanding of both the nature of the modern-day doctor–patient relationship and its association with medical power itself. It concludes by presenting palliative cancer care in general practice as a suitable framework to examine such issues. Interviews with cancer patients, their family carers, and general practitioners (GPs) provided the data upon which this book is based.

The first chapter describes the experience of cancer (or the 'cancer world') of the patient and family carer, and compares it to the cancer world of the GP. This leads to the second chapter, which studies the interaction between these different cancer worlds throughout the illness trajectory. Issues of compatibility and the prerequisites for doctor–patient harmony feature prominently.

The key threat to harmony, namely the universal issue of clinical uncertainty, is examined in the third chapter. The complexity of uncertainty and its many different forms are outlined, together with their implications for medical power and the clinical relationship. The findings suggest that the way in which uncertainty is expressed and managed might *reflect* doctor–patient compatibility instead of merely *determining* it.

The fourth chapter introduces the notions of perceived distance and ownership as deeper components of the doctor–patient relationship—components that ultimately determine its stability. In particular, the phenomenon of excessive doctor–patient closeness emphasised the instability inherent in socially constructed notions of 'doctor' and 'patient'. Such instability reached its ultimate expression in the phenomenon of role reversal. This held major implications for the nature of medical power and the doctor–patient relationship.

The fifth chapter begins by summarising the findings and systematically addressing each of the key questions posed in the Introduction. This is then used as a platform to construct the Model of Bi-Directional Care, a new model of GP–cancer patient interaction in palliative care. The book concludes by reflecting upon the implications of this model for clinical practice, research design and future health policy.

This work is written primarily for medical and nursing practitioners and students, although I am certain that medical anthropologists and sociologists will also find it useful.

The completion of a work such as this relies upon many people. I thank Dr Robyn Mary Vafiadis, Evlambia Vafiadis, Fr Spyridon, Fr Elias and my wider circle of family and friends for their constant support. I also thank the General Practice Evaluation Program (Commonwealth Government of Australia) for a three-year scholarship that enabled me to conduct this work. I am especially indebted to the people with cancer, their family carers and the GPs who went to considerable efforts to share their special worlds with me. Their support, generosity and enthusiasm was remarkable and inspirational. I was well supported in accessing families by Ms Anne Turley, Ms Noala Flynn and Ms Jo Wilson, respective directors of the

Melbourne City Mission, Mercy Hospice Care and Southport hospices. Several of my general practitioner colleagues also assisted in this task.

Two other people deserve special mention. The inspirational guidance, support and encouragement provided by Professor Allan Kellehear, Head of the Palliative Care Unit at La Trobe University, have been instrumental in the genesis of this book. Professor Kellehear's kindness and generosity have been extraordinary. I owe him an enormous amount. Professor Doris Young, Head of the Department of General Practice at the University of Melbourne, has likewise been a steadfast support. Her influence and care over many years have been very special and are treasured.

The Department of General Practice and Public Health at the University of Melbourne served as my 'headquarters' during this project. Everyone there was wonderful to work with, particularly Professor Hedley Peach, Ms Sandra Turner, Ms Alison Temperley, Dr Debbie Yarmo, Ms Colleen Nordstrom, Ms Vanessa Ho and Mr Kevin Choi. My academic colleagues in the 'Pickles Club', the Department's research support group, have also been of great assistance. I thank them as well as the resource centre of the Royal Australian College of General Practitioners in South Melbourne for providing me with many requested reference articles from the academic literature.

I deeply appreciate the work of McGraw-Hill Australia in publishing this book, particularly the efforts of Ms Meiling Voon, Ms Sybil Kesteven and Ms Frith Luton. Their courteous and professional approach has been greatly valued.

Finally, but very importantly, I thank all of my own patients for the many things they have shared with me and taught me over the years.

Introduction

An understanding of the patient's experience of illness is central to the provision of optimal medical care (McWhinney, 1989). In the clinical setting, the primary realm where such understanding is established is the doctor–patient relationship. This relationship presupposes the existence of medical authority or power (the terms here are used interchangeably), since the patient is the dependent party who potentially has an enormous amount at stake. In palliative care, this includes the patient's very self and life.

The social force and nature of medical authority has fluctuated throughout history. This Introduction examines the expression of such authority in the clinical setting. The first part analyses the socio-historical contexts that shaped the nature of the doctor–patient relationship as it exists today in the West. This offers a view of the relationship from *without*. The second part uses this as a foundation to analyse the doctor–patient relationship from *within*, examining the concept of medical power at the individual level. This will include how power is defined and understood by the main players, and the impact of clinical uncertainty and ambiguity upon it.

This review will argue that medical power itself is struggling to reconcile rational scientific methods with an emerging personal emphasis on the patient. New questions are generated about medical power and the nature of the doctor–patient relationship. The Introduction closes by outlining a framework for answering these questions, set in the field of palliative cancer care in general practice.

The social history of medical power and the doctor–patient relationship

Medicine and the doctor have not always held the eminent positions that they do today. The Hippocratic writings, Greek medical treatises compiled in the fifth and fourth centuries BC, are the earliest recorded works that *systematically* analyse and debate the nature of medicine, disease and its treatment, and medical ethics (Lloyd, 1983). Ancient Greek doctors had no legally recognised qualifications and medicine was not as distinctly defined as it is today—the boundaries between doctor, herbalist, spiritualist, midwife and gymnastic trainer were hazy at best (Lloyd, 1983). The professional position of the doctor was thus socially tenuous.

Medicine, however, gradually solidified as a distinct profession. Its interaction with philosophy helped to shape and define epistemological and methodological approaches to knowledge and reason. Such issues extended into the moral sphere. The Hippocratic Oath (Lloyd, 1983) stressed the doctor's need to always strive to help the sick and never to harm or wrong them. The concern for ethics also had *sacred* connotations concerning the need for moral perfection. The Canon in the Hippocratic Corpus comments thus on the medical art: 'Holy things are revealed only to holy men. Such things must not be made known to the profane until they are initiated into the mysteries of science' (Lloyd, 1983: 69). Healing in such a context was a sacred act that extended beyond the restoration of the body alone.

Such principles were central to the establishment of houses for the sick, poor and destitute in the early Christian era (Rosen, 1963). Although much of the care was provided by clergy and monastics, physicians also had a role in these organisations, and their example later spread to other states in the middle and far east (Rosen, 1963).

The gradual administrative secularisation of the hospital, however, changed the hospital's nature. By the end of the fourteenth century, physicians had an increasing presence in the hospital (Rosen, 1963). Additionally, by the seventeenth century, the solidifying concept of the sovereign nation (Toulmin, 1990) meant that health care for the masses, in addition to that for the rich, became politically and economically significant (Rosen, 1963). This saw the establishment of many large hospitals throughout Europe and England, heralding a fundamental change to the nature of the doctor–patient relationship.

Jewson (1976) traced such a change, beginning in Middle Ages Europe, where medical care was essentially a commodity of the rich. The high social rank of the patient conferred considerable power to them, and the diagnostic process was focused on the *patient's account of their symptoms*. During this period of 'Bedside Medicine', illness was defined 'by its external and subjective manifestations rather than its internal and hidden causes' (Jewson, 1976).

This state of affairs was changed with the advent of the large hospital in eighteenth century France. State-ownership had made possible the opening of many large hospitals, far greater in size than had been seen before (Waddington, 1973). However, poor conditions and high mortality rates led to the hospital becoming the squalid realm of the poor, while the upper classes continued to receive private care at home (Waddington, 1973). In such hospital settings, the social power-balance between doctor and patient was reversed, and now favoured the doctor. Failure to comply with suggested therapies, including invasive surgery before the advent of adequate anaesthesia, equated to instant discharge from hospital (Waddington, 1973). This climate of 'Hospital Medicine' afforded doctors unprecedented access to patients' bodies (Jewson, 1976). Greater emphasis on *examination* had shifted nosology towards *visible* changes in the body, and further from the felt experience of the patient (Jewson, 1976). The application of statistical methods in this period further enhanced this trend by defining clinical certainty as a *quantitative* phenomenon (Jewson, 1976).

Physical observation of pathological processes in the living body or the corpse in dissection, however, was confounded by illnesses that produced no visible changes to body structure (Foucault, 1994). The 'essence' of many illnesses was thus elusive (Foucault, 1994). By the mid-nineteenth century, efforts were made to define this essence through the study of cellular chemistry and physiology. In this new period of 'Laboratory Medicine', diagnosis became increasingly reliant on tests upon body tissues and fluids (Jewson, 1976). The social presence of the patient became even less necessary to the medical encounter (Kellehear, 1998), and this was further spurred by continuing advances in medical technology.

The explosion of medical knowledge (in the ensuing years in anatomy, physiology, pathology, microbiology, pharmacology and anaesthetics) greatly diversified medicine. Soon, hospitals became safe and essential places for treatment because their technology was not readily extendible to the home situation (Rosen, 1963). However, specialisation and sub-specialisation made the *homogeneous* presence of the 'complete' doctor more remote. Medicine's power into the twentieth century became a *collective* power owned by the profession as a whole, and not necessarily by the individual doctor (who was only a small part of this grander structure).

In the social sense, the *doctor*–patient relationship increasingly became the *doctors*–patient relationship, as the *option* of seeing a more experienced clinician had become readily available. This opened the potential to challenge the authority of individual doctors, especially those perceived to be positioned lower on the ladder of prestige.

Attention is now turned to behaviour at the interface between health and illness in order to derive more specific information about the place of medical power in the doctor–patient relationship.

The return of power to the patient: behaviour in health and illness

Concomitant to medicine's *collective* increase in medical power, the mid-twentieth century saw changes to how the health profession viewed the person of the patient. The 'New Public Health' movement (Kellehear, 1998) recognised the important contribution that patients themselves could make towards their own health. This gave rise to emphasis on the paradigms of health promotion and preventive medicine. The patient no longer *passively* followed medical instructions, but had a social presence and a status of *active responsibility* within the doctor–patient relationship.

The importance of patient participation in health maintenance led to intensive studies of health and illness behaviour, and to theoretical models from sociology and psychology that attempted to explain such behaviour. These included the Health Belief Model (Becker, 1979; Box I.1), the Illness Behaviour Model (Mechanic, 1968; Box I.2.), and more generalised models such the Theory of Planned Behaviour (Ajzen, 1988; Box I.3). Medical authority now had a conscious need to work *with* patients, albeit for the central purpose of enhancing patient *compliance*. If behaviour could be predicted, then it could also be potentially modified.

BOX I.1 Key elements of the Health Belief Model (after Becker, 1979)

PHASE 1	There is readiness to act against illness, depending on its perceived threat.
PHASE 2	The feasibility of a given behaviour to counteract illness is weighed up against the potential physical, social, psychological and financial costs of the behaviour.
PHASE 3	A stimulus, either internal (e.g. symptom severity) or external (e.g. influence of family) triggers execution of the health behaviour.

BOX I.2 Key elements of the Model of Illness Behaviour (after Mechanic, 1968)

1 Illness recognition	
2 Illness appraisal	
3 Health action(s)	nil
	self treat
	consult close other (e.g. family member)
	seek external help (e.g. doctor)
4 Subsequent responses	(dependent on specific illness circumstances).

BOX I.3 Ajzen's Theory of Planned Behaviour (after Ajzen, 1988)

Attitude towards the behaviour

Social acceptability of behaviour → Intention → Behaviour

Ability to perform the behaviour

Although aimed towards the collective good of the state as much as towards the individual, such attempts to understand the patient were concurrent with an evolving social change throughout the world (Toulmin, 1990). This movement desired to re-marry rational science to a compassionate view of the person, thereby beginning the dismantling of scientific rationalism. The establishment of *qualitative* method in the mid-1960s as an academically sound and rigorous research tool also greatly furthered this process.

The push to incorporate the patient's illness experience into clinical method led to a critical re-appraisal of models of health and illness behaviour. The models' attempts to understand such behaviour relied on medical and psychological definitions of 'correct' or 'ideal' behaviour (Good, 1994). They were thus tainted by rationalist and reductionist notions. The models also ignored the effects of the personal encounter with the doctor, how this affects the behaviour of both doctor and patient, and the role that medical power plays in such a process. A more specific way of examining such a context lies in a description of the doctor–patient relationship itself.

Models of the doctor–patient relationship

Parsons (1951) was among the earliest to theorise specifically about the nature of the doctor–patient relationship (see Box I.4), although his theory focused primarily on the relevance of illness to the wider social system, rather than to the individual person.

BOX I.4 Doctor and patient roles (after Parsons, 1951)

SOCIAL EXPECTATIONS OF THE SICK ROLE
1 The ill person is exempted from their normal duties.
2 The ill person needs help to become well.
3 The ill person must want to become well.
4 The ill person must seek competent help, usually from a doctor, and follow their advice.

SOCIAL EXPECTATIONS OF THE DOCTOR'S ROLE
1 The doctor has responsibility for the patient.
2 The doctor must facilitate the patient's recovery through medical science.
3 The doctor is sanctioned to have full access to the patient's body and details of their private life in order to cure the patient.
4 The doctor must be objective and focus only on the patient's interests.

Other early models of the doctor–patient relationship had similar difficulties in that they did not neatly fit the complete reality of the individual clinical consultation. Some of these models (see Box I.5) focused less on doctor and patient roles and more upon who had *control* in the doctor–patient encounter. This was an advance because it recognised that the doctor did not always have full control. However, it did not consider the effects that persons close to the patient could have upon the process of control. Nor did it describe the dynamics of control. Additionally, it did not consider that control itself may be applicable to differing aspects of the illness, and could therefore be *simultaneously* present and absent. For example, in cancer illness, pain and other symptoms might be well controlled whereas the eventual death of the patient may not be preventable.

Other models (see Box I.6) viewed the doctor–patient relationship according to how active each participant was. Although importantly demonstrating that the clinical problem *itself* shaped the relationship, this model remained simplistic and did not consider the doctor as being in anything but full control.

BOX I.5 A model of the doctor–patient relationship according to level of control (Stewart and Roter, 1981, cited in Morgan, 1991)

'Paternalism': Doctor has control
'Consumerism': Patient has control
'Mutuality': Control shared between doctor and patient
'Default': Neither doctor nor patient has control

BOX I.6 A model of the doctor–patient relationship according to level of participation (Szasz & Hollander, 1956, cited in Bloom & Wilson, 1979)

'Activity-passivity' (parent–infant model)
Doctor administers treatment, patient passively receives it (e.g. anaesthesia, acute trauma, coma).

'Guidance-cooperation' (parent–adolescent model)
Doctor instructs, patient obeys (e.g. acute infectious illness).

'Mutual participation' (adult–adult model)
Doctor helps patient to help themselves. (e.g. psychiatric counselling).

Balint's (1964) work on the general practitioner (GP)–patient relationship highlighted the importance of the patient's life circumstances to the nature of clinical encounter, and the intrinsic therapeutic value of the clinical relationship *itself*. However, this work viewed the relationship mainly from the viewpoint of the GP, not the patient. Statements on 'educating' or 'training' patients, and on the belief that 'we doctors have successfully trained our patients … to expect a routine clinical examination and to accept it without much embarrassment or apprehension' (Balint, 1964: 239, 255) all infer patient inferiority in the clinical relationship. The importance of this work, however, was its demonstration of the limitations of science alone in solving real, everyday problems. This was in harmony with Engel's (1977) 'bio-psycho-social approach' to the patient. Engel's model, however, was also rationalistic because it divided the essentially indivisible whole of the patient into neat and simple components.

All of the above models could not account for the dynamic nature of the doctor–patient relationship, that is, how it *evolved* over time. The effects of practical and social constraints (such as time limitations, cost and availability of medical services), as well as moral dilemmas (for example, contraception issues in teenage minors and euthanasia issues) were also not adequately incorporated. Such issues made the clinical relationship difficult to encompass with a theoretical model.

Instead of a model *describing* doctor–patient interaction, research emphasis gradually shifted to study how interaction was *generated* in the clinical relationship. This 'meaning-centred tradition' (Good, 1994: 52–6) highlighted mechanisms of *mutual* understanding at the *individual level* and how they could facilitate (or hinder) the clinical method. Such progress helped to rediscover the importance of systems of healing *outside* the medical establishment, where most morbidity is managed by common household and community remedies (Kleinman, 1978). Such realisations led to the term 'disease', referring to the raw pathological problem, being replaced by 'illness', which encompassed the personal impact of the disease on the patient and family (Kleinman, 1978). Similarly, 'curing' gave way to 'healing', again referring to the totality of the person instead of merely to their physical disease (Kleinman, 1978). Healing is thus possible even if cure is not, and illness is always amenable to treatment even if disease is not. New paradigms for the clinical method that reflect such progress (see boxes I.7 & I.8) represent the current 'state of the art'.

Medical power and the delivery of medical care

The trend towards a greater interest in the patient has been paralleled by social changes in the structure and delivery of medical care. In the 1960s in the United States of America, progress towards specialisation and sub-specialisation created a practical backlash regarding general access to health care, leading to a solidification of the Family Medicine movement (Kamien, 1997). Great Britain and Australia soon followed suit with more official recognition of general practice as a respectable discipline that could deal with most medical problems (Kamien, 1997). The GP thus became the 'main' doctor and 'gatekeeper' to the established medical system, emphasising *personalised* care. The impersonal *doctors*–patient relationship (p. 4) was thus

BOX I.7 Enhancing and utilising cultural awareness in clinical practice
(after Kleinman, 1978)

STEP 1	Elicit the patient's explanatory model for their illness and its impact upon them.
STEP 2	Present the medical explanatory model, comparing it to the patient's model to assess discrepancies.
STEP 3	Construct an illness problem list and negotiate a corresponding intervention for each item.
STEP 4	Clinically follow-up to assess progress in terms of 'curing' and 'healing'.
STEP 5	Teach the method to other professional colleagues.

BOX I.8 The patient-centred method (after McWhinney, 1989)

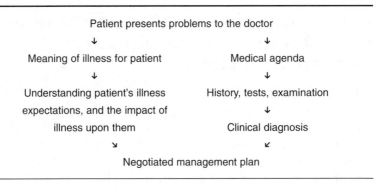

shifting back to the more personal *doctor*–patient relationship.

Such positive, patient-centred progress neutralises comments from authors like Willis (1983), who view medicine as an institution that dominates patients and allied professions such as nursing. However, the negotiation inherent in such progressive approaches has not evened up the balance entirely. Decision-making is ultimately based on an understanding of the illness that is biomedically framed. This asymmetry of knowledge between doctor and patient is unavoidable, yet serves as the foundation of the principle of informed consent (Silverman, 1987). Such asymmetry of knowledge, however, need not be considered negative. Silverman (1987), for example, has shown the importance of medical control and authority in offering confidence and comfort to families in a paediatric heart surgery unit. This also applies to less dramatic settings such as general practice (McWhinney, 1989).

In addition, knowledge is in itself only one component of power, as seen in the vulnerability and frustration felt by physicians who themselves have serious illness (see Vanderwoude, 1988). Further, could the incorporation of biopsychosocial and spiritual dimensions, implicit in patient-centred approaches, subject the patient to *excessive* scrutiny? As Silverman (1987: 189) states: 'The humane, liberating impulse sits neatly side by side with total surveillance within a clinic turned confessional. It may well be that the only way to oppose this trend is to reject the ever greater extension of the health-care team in the direction of a further range of psychological expertise.' Such a patient-centred process, because of the breadth of its scope, 'is also less explicit about its mechanisms of surveillance' compared with pathological biomedicine (Silverman, 1987: 192), and is thus harder to scrutinise and opens itself to potential abuses.

The compatibility of medical power with doctor–patient equality: current challenges

The initial question, then, of understanding how medical power influences the course of the doctor–patient relationship and the way that each experiences the illness has led into very broad frameworks of reference. Ultimately, the insurmountable problem of inequality of medical knowledge between doctor and patient confounds the idealistic pursuit of equality of power in the relationship. The existence of beneficial or necessary forms of medical power that can facilitate patients' personal control and security (Silverman, 1987; Maseide, 1991), the potentially negative 'total surveillance' of the comprehensive 'whole-patient' approach (Silverman, 1987: 189) and the fact that many doctors and patients genuinely *care* about each other (Rosser & Maguire, 1982) also confound the precise place of power within such a relationship.

In terms of the balance of power in the doctor–patient relationship, Silverman (1987) and Maseide (1991) note the importance of considering the clinical context in which this occurs (with all of its practical constraints), as well as the complex limitations of the spoken word in conveying feeling and emotion.

It seems, then, that it is the *dynamics* and the *process* of reconciling scientific rationalism with a person-centred approach that offers the best means of assessing the role and place of medical power in the doctor–patient relationship. However, such a process of reconciliation is historically very young (Toulmin, 1990) and has situated medicine awkwardly in the process of serving the needs of the individual as well as the wider community. Evidence of such awkwardness is now clearly apparent in works attempting to reconcile these paradigms, such as those studying the effects of emotion and spirituality on physical health. Here, complex phenomena are often reduced to a mathematical binomial function (for example, health effects of prayer versus no prayer) that is then analysed for statistical significance (see, for instance, Kune, Kune & Watson, 1993). And despite the general recognition of qualitative research methods, the medical literature remains saturated with mathematical calculations of chance. Skolbekken (1995) has termed this phenomenon the 'risk epidemic' and notes that it is continuing to increase.

Conversely, critiques of medical dominance (for example, Willis, 1983) fail to consider adequately the practical realities within which rational science has to be applied. The paradigms of biomedical science and the humanities are therefore presently colliding in clinical practice, rather than harmoniously intertwining. How, then, can the *doctor*–patient relationship be most efficiently reconciled to the *doctors*–patient relationship (see p. 4) given that *both* notions are clearly essential? Can they yet be compatible, and under what circumstances?

Given that it is the dynamics of *interpersonal interaction* that hold clues to such questions, it becomes necessary to focus more inwardly and narrowly on the role and person of the 'new' doctor and the 'new' patient in Western society today, both being social products of the broad movements discussed above. For the role of the 'new' doctor, the key issues relate to gender, increasing medical technology and knowledge, the issue of continuity of care, and an increased accountability to their patients and the public. For the role of the 'new' patient (or potential patient), the key issues relate to altered profiles of morbidity and mortality, better awareness and knowledge relating to health and medical matters, and expectations of high quality, participatory medical care. As will be seen, these issues actually *contribute* towards the clash between the paradigms of compassion versus hard science that have been cited above.

The 'new' doctor

The 'new' doctor in the Western world is no longer almost exclusively male, although this is a new trend, as attested by relatively recent book titles such as 'The Doctor, *His* Patient and the Illness' (Balint, 1964). Female doctors are now increasingly entering all branches of the medical workforce, especially general practice, where they are more likely to work part-time than men (Dickinson, Lalor, Calcino, Douglass & Knight, 1996). Compared with their male counterparts, their work load is often composed of longer consultations and a higher proportion of female patients (Dickinson et al., 1996). In a literature review, West (1993) found conflicting evidence on whether female doctors differed from male doctors in terms of their patient-centredness: some studies concluded that women were more caring, person-oriented doctors compared to men, while others concluded that men and women doctors do not differ in their styles of care. The point relevant to medical power is this: because gender is 'accomplished' in particular social situations, rather than being passively 'assigned' (West, 1993), and because the male–female dichotomy is used by every society to classify and socialise its members (Helman, 1990), then a changing gender composition in the medical workforce must effect changes to the way medical power is conceived and expressed. In this context, traditional views of nursing as a female institution subservient to a male medical profession might also influence public perception of the authority of female doctors. Potentially, gender may also be used bluntly, especially by male patients against female practitioners, in coercing or threatening the doctor (see also Bellamy, 1996 for a broader discussion of this topic).

Increasingly, also, the 'new' doctor has to master far more medical knowledge and technology compared with their more distant predecessors. Although offering the opportunity of consolidating medical power, this has also presented new dilemmas. Expectations of medicine's ability to cure have been *heightened*, as exemplified by the phenomenon of 'role-forcing' (Glaser & Strauss, 1965), where patients or families attempt to force the doctor to *do something* in circumstances where very little can be done. In a paradoxical way, such expectation is concurrent with the criticism of medicine's inability to heal because it is over-focused on curing. The time-honoured approach of letting nature take its course in many illnesses has thus been transformed. The pressure to prescribe antibiotic medications for viral illnesses is an example that reflects such a dilemma: the act of prescribing may be seen as a more active offer of help than a plan not involving a prescription (see McWhinney, 1989).

With advancing technology and understanding of pathophysiology, diagnosis has also been progressively pushed further back into earlier phases of illness, improving patient prognosis. Whereas in the past, for example, rectal bleeding was perceived as *the* symptom for cancer of the bowel, today emphasis has shifted toward *any* alteration in bowel habit, whether bloody or not (Kumar & Clark, 1994). Such emphasis on earlier detection, however, has increased the level of ambiguity and uncertainty associated with diagnosis, creating practical and ethical dilemmas along a number of planes. For example, *what* constitutes significant alteration in bowel habit? *When* should this be investigated? *How* and *how extensively* should it be investigated? The availability of computerised tomographic or magnetic resonance imaging scanning for diagnosis of brain tumours is similar. The critical question when confronted by a well-looking patient with a chronic headache is *who* should receive the test, *when* and under *what circumstances*? Medical advances in genetics have also extended this dilemma to the *healthy and asymptomatic* individual by establishing (often tentative) associations between genetic markers and serious illness.

The issue of how extensively to investigate is often further compounded by the potential availability of many testing procedures, all of which vary in terms of their applicability, sensitivity, specificity and physical and psychological safety to the patient (Vafiadis, 1996). The situation for treatment is also similar. Medical advances have made treatment regimens themselves complex and morally challenging, especially if they are potentially life-threatening (such as bone-marrow transplantation, aggressive chemotherapy, or invasive surgery). Other moral issues relate to equity in distribution and access to medical services, and the use of scarce life-sustaining resources, such as artificial ventilators and intensive-care unit beds.

Medical uncertainty, therefore, has been paradoxically *generated* from advancing knowledge and renewed attention to the moral duty owed to the person of the patient. Clearly, then, medical uncertainty is more complex than Fox (1957) had perceived it, because it refers to more than a lack of biomedical knowledge in the doctor or the medical corpus itself. Rather, it points to an inherent uncertainty *within* the particular clinical situation itself, including its *moral* significance.

In response to new uncertainties that have been created by advancing knowledge and technology, attempts to standardise practice to deliver the best possible care have also inadvertently subjected it to a form of regimentation that represents the antithesis of the compassionate, individualised approach. Increasingly, new forces external to the doctor–patient relationship have begun to redictate its terms in subtle ways. The advent of clinical guidelines, the preponderance of 'risk' calculations in medical literature (Skolbekken, 1995), and the rising epidemic of medical litigation (MacLennan, 1993) all attest to the considerable tension between the newly re-discovered emphasis on compassionate approaches and a persisting, more emotively straightforward and concrete rationalism. Direct threats of medico-legal repercussions have created the new and negative phenomenon of defensive medicine, which is costly, and clearly reflects a perceived vulnerability on the part of the doctor. Assault and harassment of doctors (see Bellamy, 1996) shows that such vulnerability is not only confined to their professional status and realm. Medical power may thus be more fragile than perceived.

The 'new' patient

The 'new' patient is progressively ageing due to improved public health measures, especially regarding nutrition, water quality and sanitation (Hetzel, 1982); and medical advances such as the discovery of antibiotic drugs and the development of vaccines. Average life expectancy at birth in Australia rose from 51 years for males and 54.8 years for females between 1891 and 1900 (Hetzel, 1982) to 75 years for males and 80.9 years for females in 1996 (Australian Institute of Health and Welfare, 1996). The older patient is not only relatively new to medicine, but presents differing morbidity and mortality patterns. Chronic heart and lung illness have overtaken infectious disease as the main cause of death in the Western world. In addition, most types of cancer rise in incidence with increased longevity. Increasing age is also linked to other chronic illnesses such as arthritis and strokes, which challenge medicine because they cannot be cured. That these illnesses are common and require relatively frequent medical attention also serves to magnify their clinical challenge.

The new patient is also generally more health conscious and preoccupied with maintaining good health. Examples of this heightened health consciousness include the emphasis on healthy eating and weight control; the aerobics fitness movement; increased emphasis on workplace safety; the prohibition of tobacco advertisements; and the growing movement to ban cigarette smoking in public places.

Passive exposure to information technology, and the ability to actively access it, are also relatively novel hallmarks of the new patient which have greatly enhanced awareness of health issues. These, in turn, generate demand for more information. Outside of the formal education system, a key source of information is television, especially its news reports, talk shows, documentaries and medically based series and soap operas. Other important information sources include the print media (such as newspapers and popular magazines), radio, and the telephone service. The recent growth of the world-wide electronic web or 'internet' has also ensured that the computer has become a prominent tool in accessing and utilising health information.

This enormous exposure to health information does not ignore, but rather actively covers, more negative issues including medical errors and medical malpractice and litigation. This heightens suspicion against doctors and reinforces the reality of their fallibility. Coexistent information on consumer rights, legal services and advocacy therefore also preoccupies the 'new' patient, illustrating their somewhat paradoxical relationship with medicine. Shorter (1985: 211) has summarised this paradox by stating that 'although people (today) … are far more sensitive to symptoms and more willing to seek care for them than ever before', their '… signs of alienation from the medical profession … sets the stage for a crisis'. A growing public interest in alternative and complementary medicine is a consequence of this phenomenon (Shorter, 1985).

All of this has served to change the 'new' patient's perception of themselves. The 'new' patient has reacted against the impersonal and insensitive aspects of scientific medicine and is also aware of its inability to deal adequately with all health concerns, but simultaneously respects its many achievements. This has altered the nature of the new patient's self-identity in their encounters with mainstream medicine. Although still yielding themselves to medicine, the 'new' patient exhibits what Goffman (1961, cited in Kellehear & Fook, 1989) has termed 'role-distancing', sometimes preferring to be called a 'client' or a 'consumer' rather than a 'patient'. This may be a reaction designed to prevent loss of self during chronic or severe illness (Charmaz, 1983).

Statement of the problem

In summary, the conception of medical power as a largely negative, dominating force has confused its function, place and influence in the clinical setting. It has also, therefore, confused a proper understanding of the nature of the doctor–patient relationship. Medical power is clearly a complex phenomenon that is both framed and expressed according to broad social and cultural norms beyond the individual control of either doctor or patient, as well as particular factors within and personal interaction between doctor, patient and significant others. Within the interpersonal interaction, the term 'power' can only be effectively analysed when considered in relation to its *intent*, something which the sociological and medical literature has underemphasised. The significance of this is apparent if one considers, as an example, that even the patient-centred approach is capable of being applied mechanically rather than sensitively. In other words, the patient-centred approach is *forced* if applied mechanically, and *genuine* if applied sensitively.

The review to this point has defined several issues that need clarification in order to understand the doctor–patient relationship and how each person experiences the illness. These issues are not mutually exclusive, but rather mutually influence each other.

How 'patient-centred' is the patient-centred approach?

Critiques of the patient-centred approach suggest that it may represent an expression of medical power itself, rather than being exclusively empowering for the patient (Silverman, 1987). Is this so, and if it is, how empowering is the actual process for the patient? Is the attainment of patient empowerment itself *dependent* upon the medical power implicated by such methods? These questions probe the blurry links between 'power', 'control', 'knowledge' and 'competence' which are critical for a more thorough understanding of this area (Maseide, 1991; Adamson, 1997).

Medical power has different forms that must be more clearly differentiated

Medical power can be both desirable as well as undesirable, and its expression may be forceful and obvious or subtle and imperceptible, according to the situation. This raises questions as to the nature of differing forms of medical power, how they are expressed and received, how they relate to each other, and their ability to coexist. Silverman (1987) observed strategies of medical power in different specialist outpatient clinics, however, less controlled and more common or routine settings need further study.

The influence of medical power upon the medical profession itself is unclear

The existence of a medical hierarchy ensures that the force of medical power is not only conveyed from doctor to patient but also from doctor to doctor. Apart from being directly conveyed, such hierarchical pressure may also manifest *internally*, within the doctor, because it shapes their own medical expectations of themselves. The impact that this has upon the *individual* doctor–patient relationship is unclear.

The interplay between medical power and clinical and moral uncertainty needs further investigation

Clinical and moral uncertainty directly confound medical power and have the potential to erode confidence. Moral uncertainty may also be linked to a tension between professional association versus personal friendship in the doctor–patient relationship, a tension which may be facilitated by patient-centred approaches and which has further implications related to medical power. How such issues are managed, and their effects on the doctor–patient relationship, need clarification.

Circumstances, methods and consequences of challenges to medical power need clarification

Medical power is not absolute but may be challenged in many different ways, ranging from the implicit (as in non-compliance or gentle questioning of medical actions) to the explicit (as in litigation). Is medical authority inversely proportional to patient authority? When is medical power challenged and under what circumstances? What prompts such challenges and what is their effect? How great a role do structural constraints, such as limited consultation times, contribute? What role does the discrepancy between the *actual* versus the *perceived* potential of medical power play? Also, because doctors themselves are subject to the force of medical power, do they *themselves* challenge it, and how?

Issues of the permanence or reversibility of the effects of power remain unclear

Progress through the illness has the potential to alter the status or the degree of medical power. For example, complications arising from therapy might see medical power progress from respected to criticised. Other situations may see the converse, where medical power increases from initial criticism to final appreciation. Although relevant in shaping the therapeutic relationship, the *permanence* or *reversibility* of the effects of previous statuses of power remain unclear.

This book will focus on the issues of how medical power relates to, is reconciled with, and is affected by clinical and moral uncertainty and progressive deterioration in incurable illness. The nature of this task demands a comparison of medical and non-medical viewpoints. The key issues will be studied in relation to their effects on the *stability* of doctor and patient roles over time, and to their effects on the *identity* of both doctor and patient. This is expected to shed further insight into the nature of the patient-centred approach and to contribute towards a better understanding of clinical method and its application.

A framework for examining issues of authority in the doctor–patient relationship

Ultimately it is the 'interpersonal' level of interaction that gives meaning to and influences how the 'structural' components are perceived and experienced (Kellehear, 1994). It is at the individual level, then, in all its complexity, that a more complete understanding is to be reached (Good, 1994). Individual experience, however, must be placed within a framework that will optimise the pursuit of the key questions that have been posed. The framework chosen here is *palliative cancer care* delivered through *general practice*, and bridging *cross-cultural experiences*. Some brief comments on each of these realms should help to further clarify their relevance.

Palliative cancer care

Palliative care offers a relevant context for examining medical power because the primary source of medical authority, namely the ability to cure, is missing. The emphasis on 'total care' of patient and family (Woodruff, 1993) in highly emotive settings poses a strong challenge to the health professional. The need for ongoing medical contact (and indeed *frequent* contact due to unstable illness states) poses two further difficulties. The first is the intrusion upon the private and intimate aspects of people's lives and bodies, which challenges patient and family alike. The second is that attending health professionals are *repeatedly* confronted by progressive illness, with all of its inherent difficulties and uncertainties.

Cancer is especially relevant because it is relatively common. Advances in treatment which prolong survival may impair quality of life because of side-effects or simply through increasing the already stressful time left to live. Issues of autonomy and control are implicit here. Cancer, however, is also potentially curable or at least amenable to effective, useful palliation. Such a potential *multiplicity of outcomes* offers a range of different contexts from which power, control and the illness experience might be examined.

The general practice setting

Generally, trends are increasing for palliative care, and also death itself, to occur in the home setting (Woodruff, 1993). In the Australian health system this places the GP at the centre of such care, a position often favoured by the general public and by patients (Charlton, 1991). Although it confers authority to the GP, it also carries considerable responsibility and vulnerability. The practical necessity of a close-knit multidisciplinary approach, for example, potentially exposes the GP to the effects of medical power emanating from colleagues who are also involved in the patient's care. In addition, cancer challenges the GP by touching upon their own sense of mortality. This challenge is enhanced by the likelihood of their close familiarity with the patient and family. Symptom control, although generally possible and effective in the home setting, can also be difficult.

Structurally, home care also 'sandwiches' the GP between the lived reality of the illness in the community and the more concrete, biomedical philosophy of the tertiary hospital which has trained them. The direct relationship, of belonging and mediation between the philosophy of these two very different worlds can create considerable stresses (Rosser & Maguire, 1982). Additionally, when all contacts are home-based in advanced illness, the GP works away from the security of their own surgery.

Cross-cultural experiences

To date much of the discussion has focused upon how medical culture became differentiated and alienated from the culture of general society. General society, however, is itself culturally diverse. In Australia in 1988, twenty-five per cent of the population was of non-Anglo-Celtic descent, sixty per cent of the population had at least two different ethnic origins, and over two million Australians spoke a language other than English (Ferguson & Browne, 1991). This is paralleled by a wide cultural diversity in the composition of the Australian medical and allied health workforce (National Health Strategy, 1993). Such diversity is not dissimilar in many other areas of the world. The central influence of culture upon the illness experience (Helman, 1990) makes it a key issue in medical power and doctor–patient relationships. Nowhere more than in the emotion-laden context of palliative care is the potential for contrast in cultural attitudes expected to be greater.

Examining medical authority and doctor and patient roles from particular cultural viewpoints might provide broad, 'culture-specific' details about how medical power is influenced and expressed. However, the pursuit of such details in their own right is *not* an objective of this work. Instead, the study of both *contrasts and similarities* in the experiences of different cultural groups will be used to heighten and enrich the *broader* understanding of medical power in the clinical relationship. It is these wider and more generally applicable ramifications that this cross-cultural component seeks to inform.

Two ethnic cultures, Anglo-Celtic and Greek, are considered. The Anglo-Celtic culture was chosen because of its size and the presence of a vast amount of literature on dying, cancer and loss that specifically relates to this culture. The Greek culture was chosen for three reasons: there is a relatively large Greek community in Australia with high prevalence in Melbourne (Hugo & Maher, 1995), where the study was based; this group has poor fluency in English compared with other ethnic groups (Hugo & Maher, 1995), which is expected to influence the illness experience and the process of care; and the author has a Greek background and fluency in Greek, which facilitated access and understanding of this community.

Implementation of the research framework

The examination of medical authority in the contexts of palliative cancer care, general practice and cross-cultural experience was conducted through the use of in-depth interviews. Cancer patients, their carers, and general practitioners provided the information on which the rest of this book is based (see Appendix for further details).

Conclusion: towards the cancer experience

In outlining the complex nature of medical authority, this Introduction has argued that the best way of understanding it is from *within* the context of the clinical relationship. Key questions concerning medical power have been presented, and a framework for answering those questions has been constructed. The first chapter will begin this task by describing the cancer worlds of patients, carers and GPs. This will define the emotional landscape of the book and will establish the analysis of the dynamic interaction between these key players.

1

Illness through the eyes of patient and doctor

The study of the doctor–patient relationship in palliative cancer care demands a mapping of the emotional context or 'landscape' of such care. Here, such a landscape refers to the entire, *lived* experience of cancer: the cancer world. This chapter describes this lived experience in two separate sections.

The first section outlines the cancer world of the patient and carer, aiming to capture the impact and the essence of the illness upon their lives. Patients and carers formed the true 'insiders' (Minichiello, Aroni, Timewell & Alexander, 1990) that *continually* and *most intimately* lived with cancer. Their world was dominated by the task of coming to terms with the illness, and the changing concept of self that cancer produced (Charmaz, 1983). There was also often a tension between an unavoidable dependence on the medical profession versus a yearning to lead a 'normal' life.

The second section examines cancer illness as it was lived by the GP. This world was dominated by the therapeutic emphasis, which continually challenged, sometimes frustrated, and yet often rewarded the doctor. Although medical treatments were framed largely in accordance with the biomedical model, they were subject to negotiation with patients and families. This facilitated a certain *flexibility* in terms of how doctors understood and executed treatment. Ways in which GPs understood and approached the management process are discussed in relation to the stage of illness progression.

The cancer experience was an *individually unique* phenomenon that altered and *evolved* over time. Therefore, in describing the cancer life or world of patients, their carers and GPs, this chapter incorporates the *range* of observed experiences, presenting a broad 'emotional overview' of the cancer experience.

The cancer world of patient and carer

Initial responses to being interviewed about cancer illness differed between Greek and Anglo-Celtic families. Many of the former group did not see the need for a formal interview. In their eyes, the situation was straightforward and obvious: they had cancer, and that said it all. What more was there to say? This reflected a generally more concrete, fatalistic outlook that many Greek informants shared about cancer. Anglo-Celtic informants were usually more ready to participate, displaying more trust and far less caution; they were more familiar and comfortable with the interview process.

Global reactions to cancer both among Greeks and Anglo-Celtics were, as expected, generally negative. However, sometimes cancer had more positive associations. Basic perceptions of cancer were also heavily influenced by the events particularly at diagnosis, and also subsequent phases of the illness. 'Pre-illness' perceptions of cancer continually evolved in parallel with events throughout the illness to determine the emotional response to it. The different emphases that were given to cancer by those interviewed are summarised thematically in Box 1.1, but not in any order of ascendancy. These were *not* mutually exclusive and could be *simultaneously* present or absent in varying combinations, or vary in emphasis at different stages of the illness.

BOX 1.1 Patient and carer emphases on cancer

Cancer as taboo	Cancer as disease and non-self
Cancer as interaction	Cancer as loss
Cancer as gain	Cancer as struggle
Cancer as self	Cancer as uncertain or unknown
Cancer as a test	Cancer as a determined outcome

Cancer as taboo

Cancer often produced feelings of anxiety and gloom. It was commonly seen as an unknown entity that generally led to death. That was consistent with widespread metaphors for cancer as discussed by Sontag (1978), such as it being a killer, a death sentence. Even the mere mention of the word 'cancer' was an 'off-limits' activity for patient and carer alike:

CYNTHIA Well when it started, when he [i.e. Simon] came in and told me, he came up to me in the hallway so he told it to me. And I just … cancer just goes through me like [clicks fingers]. You can't really say the word. I couldn't at first. And I just said to him, "Put it in the hands of the Lord". It [i.e. the previous statement] just come out … You're in shock, you're in shock for a few days, quite a few days, you sort of go in and, I think its denial. You say, "He's gonna be all right". You've got to think positive.

[Simon, age 64 with lymphoma; Cynthia, age 52—wife; Anglo-Celtic]

Whereas Simon and Cynthia had acclimatised to their illness over time, so that, according to Cynthia " … *you [can] say cancer now, I mean, back then you couldn't really say it*" *[Simon, age 64 with lymphoma; Cynthia, age 52—wife; Anglo-Celtic]*, the impression with the Greek informants was that the term 'cancer' engendered a more lasting taboo that was harder to get used to. Therefore, the word 'cancer' was often totally avoided, as one GP noted:

THEODORE We do not talk [emphasised] about the word 'cancer'. [It is referred to as] "that [emphasised] illness, … you know, doctor". "O, cancer you say?! Oh!! …" [spoken in Greek; bangs hand on table, imitating the superstition of knocking on wood to avert something bad from happening].   *[Theodore, GP, age 63; Greek]*

Such conceptions conveyed a sinister side to cancer. Sontag (1978) also noted this in her comparison of cancer to an acute myocardial infarction or other serious forms of heart disease: the latter, although just as lethal as cancer, evoked less emotional fear or terror. Such negative images of cancer extended to the medical profession by reminding doctors of their own mortality:

BEN Well I know personally that I am vulnerable to seeing … a wasting process. … I find that it's, it's a threatening thing. I find the, the terror and the fear that accompanies … certain illnesses are very threatening. … And certainly they're feelings that I make a point of trying to deal with, recognise and deal with.

[Ben, GP, age 49; Jewish]

Although cancer threatened the GP informants, its prevalence made them more familiar with it compared with patient and carer informants.

Cancer was thus less mysterious for GPs. The rigorous demands for practical intervention also seemed to help them divert their focus away from the anxiety-causing aspects of cancer, and therefore to view the illness in more objective, clinical terms:

> **ANDREW** How do I deal with it? ... It's certainly very intense when you're dealing with people like this. I think it certainly makes you feel depressed. ... [pause] I guess I cope with it because it's not me, it's not my family although ... it's your patient and you do get to know them so well, especially in the palliative care situation you get really close to them ... I guess I try not to get too emotional in that sense of ... being personally involved. I tried to be detached so I can still be objective and do the right thing in terms of medical problems, and I don't think I have any difficulty in handling that. *[Andrew, GP, age early 40s; Greek]*

And again:

> **ANDREW** ... I certainly do feel low after I come out of such a place or such a house. ... But then I try ... not to dwell on it ... and not to be thinking of it all the time. ... There is that detached feeling I think ... , the fact that, "This person is going to die, thank goodness it's not me". ... There is that in it, definitely. I mean, it's not a pleasant thought but I think you have to divorce yourself somehow.
> *[Andrew, GP, age early 40s; Greek]*

Viewing cancer in a somewhat detached way made it more objective for the GP and broke down its taboo status, thereby empowering the GP to continue with the medical management. This process of 'objectification' paralleled the notion of viewing cancer as 'disease' rather than 'illness', and in so doing *opposed* the theoretical call of the literature to do the opposite—that is, to view cancer as 'illness' rather than 'disease' (see Introduction, p. 8). Stepping back a little was *not* tantamount to disregarding the presence of the patient, and some level of detachment was actually appreciated by patients and carers:

> **ALAN** ... you feel that he [the oncologist] is feeling for you and yet he doesn't get out of control. ... I don't know what happens when he goes home to his wife [laughs] but certainly when he's in his surgery he remains in control, ... which, if we're having trouble coping, that's a bit helpful. ... We don't have to help him cope with his problems too [laughs], there's only one of us that ... is in trouble.
> *[Monica, age 48 with breast cancer; Alan, age late 50s—husband; Anglo-Celtic]*

Cancer as disease and non-self

Metaphors abound of cancer as a disease that is distinctly 'non-self', as highlighted by Sontag (1978: 67): 'In cancer, non-intelligent ("primitive", "embryonic", "atavistic") cells are multiplying, and you are being replaced by the non-you.' Likewise in this study, patients, carers and GPs described cancer most often by terms that referred to it as a component of *non-self*, something foreign:

MARIA ... It had manifested like a small ... chickpea ...
> *[Maria, age 69 with breast cancer; Peter, age 74—husband; Greek];*

MARIA ... he realised what I had ...
> *[Maria, age 69 with breast cancer; Peter, age 74—husband; Greek];*

MARIA ... the sickness is a little difficult ...
> *[Maria, age 69 with breast cancer; Peter, age 74—husband; Greek];*

CHARLES ... I had a growth in the ..."
> *[Charles, age 72 with prostate cancer; Amanda, age 72—wife; Anglo-Celtic];*

MARY ... and this thing came upon us ...
> *[Panteleimon, age 62 with lung cancer; Mary, age 63—wife; Greek];*

ALAN ... it broke out again last year ...
> *[Monica, age 48 with breast cancer; Alan, age late 50s—husband; Anglo-Celtic];*

ALAN ... another ... cancer on the loose again ...
> *[Monica, age 48 with breast cancer; Alan, age late 50s—husband; Anglo-Celtic];*

and

... the tumour ...   *[used in numerous texts].*

This *'foreign-ness'* made cancer analogous to an infectious disease or other related process where the source of the problem was external and unrelated to the body itself. As non-self, cancer facilitated the strategic planning against its demise, both in medical and non-medical minds. In conjunction with the notion of *'foreign-ness'*, the cancer process was often viewed as a *destructive* one that hampered normal body functioning:

MARIA ... they told me that the bone was being eaten away, ...

[Maria, age 69 with breast cancer; Peter, age 74—husband; Greek];

MARIA ... the bone was ready to go, the cancer had started to take root, to come outside ...

[Maria, age 69 with breast cancer; Peter, age 74—husband; Greek];

FIELD NOTES ... to see her husband "melting away" in front of her was extremely difficult ...

[George, age mid-50s with lung cancer; Katerina, age ?—wife; Greek].

The perception of cancer as destructive presented major challenges to the health-care process even at seemingly innocuous points. One hospice, for example, noted that the son of Panteleimon *[Panteleimon, age 62 with lung cancer; Mary, age 63—wife; Greek]*, in his early twenties, became stressed when used by the hospital as an interpreter for his non-English speaking parents. The difficulty was not in his ability to interpret but rather that it placed him too emotionally close to such a stressful and devastating process.

Such notions of cancer as foreign and malevolent set the context for understanding the often high hopes that families placed on positive aspects of treatment. Even in cancer that was expected to progress, attaining remission (or at least arresting the rapidity of progress) lent considerable hope and emotional reprieve to families.

When it came to balancing popular metaphor against objective knowledge, the level of biological understanding of cancer was seen to vary considerably among families. Often cancer was only understood as a destructive process on a *basic level,* founded on personal observations and general medical information. Some views were simple yet accurate, such as cancer being like a weed growing out of control in the garden— although it was removable, it could spring up again *[Dimitri; Barbara, age 48 with cervical cancer; Dimitri, age 53—husband; Greek]*. Only one informant, Monica *[Monica, age 48 with breast cancer; Alan, age late 50s— husband; Anglo-Celtic]*, the most educated and professionally qualified informant, had detailed understanding of cancer's actual biology.

Cancer as interaction

Although cancer was the core medical problem, at times it was *not* the primary referent in the discussion of the illness experience. Sometimes, the discussion focused on the *interaction* with the medical and allied health system that the cancer had necessitated:

PETER It is not a few years—we have been tormented now for six years with [seeing] the doctors.

[Maria, age 69 with breast cancer; Peter, age 74—husband; Greek]

Given that Maria *[Maria, age 69 with breast cancer; Peter, age 74—husband; Greek]* had achieved excellent sustained palliation from the medical viewpoint, this suggested that the *process* of treatment was sometimes as fatiguing as the diagnosis itself.

Often, interactions with the medical system were *positive*, as with Katerina *[George, age mid-50s with lung cancer; Katerina, age ?—wife; Greek]*. The quality of her husband's home care far exceeded the care that her ill mother received in an Athens hospital for advanced cancer. In Athens, the relatives had to administer basic care to the hospitalised patient, which made her husband's care seem far more organised and thorough by comparison. That everything possible was being done, together with her religious faith, greatly assisted her own coping.

A feeling of closeness between doctor and patient also contributed to very positive interaction even in the presence of advanced illness, as noted by a GP whose patient had end-stage disseminated prostate cancer:

ANDREW ... he was actually quite an interesting person and ... once you got to know him he was really warm and friendly. He enjoyed it when I came around. ... He liked to talk. He'd get his wife to make me a coffee and a cake, you know. ... He would want to get all his sort of medical business out the way so we could sit down and have a little bit of a talk. ... I found that really, really good from my point of view.

[Andrew, GP, age early 40s; Greek]

Sometimes, however, medical interactions were not smooth, because patient or family expectations differed from medical expectations and approaches. The often frequent medical contact required by ill people enhanced such tensions and actually threatened the stability of the relationships:

ELIZABETH ... She was attending Peter Mac [a cancer hospital] regularly, every couple of months initially and then it spaced out to every six months. And then she came to me with her daughter, and this is where things deteriorated because her daughter became very involved, very pushy, wanted to know what was going

on at *all* [emphasis on the last word] times, ... wanted to question every judgment
that I was making ...   *[Elizabeth, GP, age 32; Croatian]*

Sometimes the primary focus of discussion was on how otherwise
routine modes of interaction were *altered* by the cancer. Sometimes there
was an inability between close family members to freely interact, as seen
with Simon and Cynthia *[Simon, age 64 with lymphoma; Cynthia, age 52—
wife; Anglo-Celtic]*, who could not easily discuss cancer. Sometimes there
was a desire to conceal loss of function or pain from others, as with
Charles *[Charles, age 72 with prostate cancer; Amanda, age 72—wife; Anglo-
Celtic]*, who concealed his metastatic bone pain from his wife. Sometimes
there was even a desire to conceal loss from oneself, as with Barbara
[Barbara, age 48 with cervical cancer; Dimitri, age 53—husband; Greek], who
initially ascribed her frequent vaginal bleeding to over-work rather than
potentially serious illness.

The notion of *excessive support* also proved an important one and
pointed to the patient and family's need for a balance between support
and rest or privacy:

> **MONICA** ... the hospital were lovely when I was there. Alan and the kids could
> come in at any time. They were also very good at, ... at fending off too many
> visitors or saying, "Just two or three minutes" ... so the support from them was
> terrific.
>
> *[Monica, age 48 with breast cancer; Alan, age late 50s—husband; Anglo-Celtic]*

Cancer as loss

Not infrequently, conversations centred *not* on the notion that cancer itself
was something foreign, but rather that it *induced* something foreign—an
altered life characterised by a series of *losses*:

> **MICHAEL** ... it devastated me because of, of the loss. ... I suppose it might have
> been selfish of me or whatever, but it was for the both of us. ... This was going to
> be it now, you know. Like I was right [with my own health] and we were just going
> to enjoy ourselves, you know, ...
>
> *[Clare, age 65 with stomach cancer; Michael, age 67—husband; Anglo-Celtic]*

Loss itself was a complex phenomenon because it touched on many
different realms, including the physical, emotional/psychological, social,
and spiritual/existential. Charmaz (1983) has suggested that loss of self

though altered roles and self-perception posed the greatest personal threat to the individual. Such core issues relating to the personal constitution and identity were also echoed by the informants here. For example:

MARIA ... [I didn't know] what would happen to me, or whether I would be in pain, or whether I would be *lost* [emphasis added, not actual] ...
[Maria, age 69 with breast cancer; Peter, age 74—husband; Greek]

Losses in some form and to some degree were universal. Losses were often so painful that many informants shed tears during the interviews. However, losses were weighted differently according to the particular circumstances of the individual, including their age, general satisfaction with life and personal achievements, and the nature and availability of supports. The type of cancer, its extent and rapidity of progress were also important. The *loss of mental faculties* was a particularly potent threat to the self that was emphasised in interviews with several informants, Greek and Anglo-Celtic alike. One informant put it thus:

CHARLES ... the main thing as long as nothing affects my mind, as long as my mind's working I don't mind, but if I get to the stage where I'm going to be a vegetable I most certainly don't want to stick around.
[Charles, age 72 with prostate cancer; Amanda, age 72—wife; Anglo-Celtic]

Losses could also be *actual* or *potential*. With the cancer diagnosis, potential or anticipated loss could be overwhelming before it actually eventuated, as seen with Panteleimon *[Panteleimon, age 62 with lung cancer; Mary, age 63—wife; Greek]*, who prematurely confined himself to bed after being diagnosed with lung cancer. *Uncertainty* about future progress added to such fear. Panteleimon's surrender devastated his family because in essence he wasted several weeks in bed when he could have more effectively utilised the time:

FIELD NOTES ... Mary said that he rarely got up from the time that he learned the diagnosis, but rather withdrew into himself and lost interest and enthusiasm for life. He barely got up out of bed when he was able, and at present is ... too weak to do so.
[Panteleimon, age 62 with lung cancer; Mary, age 63—wife; Greek]

Often, the *minimisation of loss* was of more central importance than the presence of the tumour itself. For example, Simon *[Simon, age 64 with lymphoma; Cynthia, age 52—wife; Anglo-Celtic]* could emotionally tolerate the presence of a lymphoma nodule on his elbow after chemotherapy, because his symptom control was reasonable:

> **INTERVIEWER** ... Are you happy to have that there?
> **SIMON** Well naturally I'm not happy, but it's not doing anything. It doesn't seem to be interfering with any other organs. It, it's in a place there that it, it can be removed surgically so ...
> **INTERVIEWER** ... you've got that one under control more or less ...
> **SIMON** Yeah, well that's ... what Dr Adams said, ... "It's not worrying you is it?". I said, "It's not worrying me, it's a bit of a nuisance but ...".
> *[Simon, age 64 with lymphoma; Cynthia, age 52—wife; Anglo-Celtic]*

Evidence to further strengthen this notion came from commentaries during which the illness was quiescent, but not absent. These showed that happiness was possible during such periods, because *hope* was enkindled for prolonged remission or cure:

> **PAULA** ... the truth is ... because he had become well we weren't expecting him to become worse. ... With the radiotherapy that he had and everything stopped for quite a considerable period, and we thought that it had stopped for [good] ... But ... in the beginning the doctor said that he might go for five years, fifteen years ...
> *[Aristotle, age 79 with prostate cancer; Paula, age ?—daughter; Greek]*

Even a fleeting quiescence could last long enough to induce feelings of renewed hope. That, however, could also create a kind of torment when deterioration followed soon after:

> **MARY** ... to see your person dying [spoken in a reflective mood] ... Sometimes I see him and cut off all my hopes, sometimes I see him and I say, "Ah, he doesn't have anything, he is good now". ... This is it. ... This is the agony now.
> *[Panteleimon, age 62 with lung cancer; Mary, age 63—wife; Greek]*

The assessment of loss was thus potentially very fluid and *relative* to the perceptions and hopes of the observer. In the case of Maria *[Maria, age 69 with breast cancer; Peter, age 74—husband; Greek]*, loss was minimised by actually *making* the diagnosis of cancer, because that at least explained her hitherto mysterious and severe symptomatology, confirmed her suspicions of cancer, and opened the way for effective symptom control. It actually induced a sense of relief.

Although cancer was often seen as a death sentence, people *resisted loss* in their attempts to normalise or stabilise. Such resistance occurred through simple hope and observation (as seen above with Mary *[Panteleimon, age 62 with lung cancer; Mary, age 63—wife; Greek]*), or through more elaborate and rationalised conceptions:

> **MONICA** ... I guess, since I've had these outbreaks, my sense is that ... I'll be very lucky if it's ... something else that gets me rather than the cancer. And, and that when I was so sick and when I was so depressed, ... particularly when I first came home, I really wished I'd gone, ... that I'd died, and didn't have to undergo the fight back. But you know, now I feel very positive about it, the fact that I can have good quality of life and be around for the kids. ... And ... I mean April is ... fifteen in December, and my big goal is to be well enough for her twenty-first. You know, I think that's a reasonable goal ... and I mean if I'm well enough for her twenty-first there's a damn good chance that I could be well for a lot longer. ... But I'm setting that as a ... as a goal ... in the knowledge that if I can survive for that number of years ... you know, another six years, then my chances for surviving for another ten after that are infinitely better than my chances of surviving for ten today.
>
> *[Monica, age 48 with breast cancer; Alan, age late 50s—husband; Anglo-Celtic]*

The need to resist loss was often crucial for daily functioning and maintenance of emotional *control*, so much so that even well organised families sometimes had no clear-cut plans for the future, approaching it on a day-by-day basis.

GPs were also subject to considerable effects related to loss, either actual or anticipated. Because many cancers were located beyond the bounds of medical cure, the loss that many doctors felt did not usually hold strong implications for their medical *ability*. (The exceptions were situations where a good prognosis was expected but not actually realised, or where symptom palliation was unexpectedly difficult.) More commonly, GPs felt sadness over the deterioration and loss of persons that they liked and had come to know well:

> **THEODORE** ... after you've been around for forty years, a lot of the patients are close. ... In fact I've known them longer than their own children have known them because I can go back four generations. They're ... I mean ... in forty years it was the great grandmother even. I go sometimes to the cemeteries and have a look at their names and think, "Oh, you know, ... there are four or five generations we're talking about. It's been a long time." ... So this closeness is very close and ... you

have a bit of a cry for a few seconds and then get back to it. ...

[Theodore, GP, age 63; Greek]

Such feelings could also be projected into the future in regard to currently healthy patients:

ANASTASIA ... I actually worry about some of my patients now who are well who are in their eighties who I'm attached to 'cause I've been seeing them for two years ... and [they] have been well and I think, "Gosh, you know, in the next five years someone's gonna die", ... And ... that's probably worse off I reckon, in a way, 'cause a lot of the palliative patients [that I now have] I've only known them as palliative patients [i.e. there was no pre-existing relationship before the terminal illness was diagnosed]. You know what I mean?

[Anastasia, GP, age 31; Greek]

Cancer as gain

Although serious illnesses such as tuberculosis have been widely romanticised in English literature and theatre, the scope for any such positive associations with cancer has been perceived as non-existent: 'Tuberculosis was an ambivalent metaphor—both a scourge and an emblem of refinement. Cancer was never viewed other than as a scourge ...' (Sontag, 1978: 61).

However, as seen across all informants, the cancer diagnosis under favourable circumstances (such as effective symptom control) could result in *gains* of various kinds. These included the facilitation of rewarding new relationships and friendships with health-care providers or other patients, or the heightening of religious awareness and spiritual contentment. The struggle to minimise loss heightened the appreciation of many positive factors in life, both by patient, family and GP. Such factors were often relatively 'simple', concomitant to the shrinking realm of function and interaction caused by progressive illness. Michael *[Clare, age 65 with stomach cancer; Michael, age 67—husband; Anglo-Celtic]*, for example, stated that although his wife Clare was greatly weakened by advanced stomach cancer, she still gained considerable satisfaction when she tested her ability to walk the length of the room and found that she could (just) do it. Barbara and Dimitri *[Barbara, age 48 with cervical cancer; Dimitri, age 53—husband; Greek]* were thankful that, even though Barbara's cancer was advanced, she had improved enough after treatment to be physically able to wash the dishes and thereby resume one of her usual, though perhaps more mundane, roles. The resumption of that familiar role kept open her links with normality and therefore her 'usual' self.

Families were often brought closer to each other and to the patient on account of the patient's illness. Relatives who had not spoken to each other in years were now doing so, and time was appreciated more and utilised more efficiently, to its maximum potential. Relatively positive progress (even though minor, such as the ability to eat a little more food to combat a wasting process), simple social interactions, and well-wishes and gestures made by others were all often magnified in the eyes of the patient and family:

> **MONICA** ... I have a faith and we are practising Christians and I feel as if it will be all right whatever happens. ... Well, I've found it very supportive that we have St Mary's Anglican in North Melbourne ... and Peter has brought me ... brought me Communion regularly when I wasn't well enough to go to church. ... And umm, my friend, who is also a chaplain where I was working, ... has called very regularly ... so with each of them there has been regular formal prayer, more formal prayer. ... But, I've just been amazed that, how many of the huge number of letters and things I've received said that, "We're praying for you". And, I mean it's a world-wide thing too, ... one of our managers is a Jehovah's Witness, ... another of our managers, the Pakistan one, is a practising Muslim, and our partner in Pakistan, you know, sent back the message when he went to Mecca earlier this year, ... "I prayed for you at Mecca." ... [They are] ... people who believe in one God, ... albeit their roots may be different ... to mine, but I've, I've really appreciated it, and it has felt ... just that I'm part of something much bigger, much, much bigger. It is a support.
>
> *[Monica, age 48 with breast cancer; Alan, age late 50s—husband; Anglo-Celtic]*

In the clinical setting this underlined the importance of supportive interventions and social support (even if hope for cure was not present), no matter how trivial such intervention might seem to an external observer:

> **ANASTASIA** ... I would go and ... see her every day, see ... if her symptoms were well controlled ... And sometimes all I did was just walk with her. ... And she said, "Oh, I feel like getting out of bed and having a walk", and ... sometimes that's all I did, and just have a chat; ...   *[Anastasia, GP, age 31; Greek]*

The reflective mood around life, death, existence and destiny that palliative care generated within GPs also often transformed their experience of care and imparted positive spiritual undertones to it. Directly continuing her line of speech from above, Anastasia remarked:

> **ANASTASIA** ... but I was, it was a good experience sort of spiritually as well ... [but] the difficulty was, you know, ... [pause] her death and ... not knowing where the barriers are, where you are a GP and where you are a friend. You know, 'cause you sort of ... grieve as well. ... And that was a bit difficult I think. ... But the family ... every year, like Christmas, I always get a card and some flowers ... it's just wonderful and ... you know ... they had a grandson who was being christened and they rang up and said, "Yeah, can you come to the christening tomorrow?". I said, "No I can't", you know [laughs], "but thank you". But, you know, really feeling part of ... really feeling as if ... you know, part of, of really being a GP, a really family GP.   *[Anastasia, GP, age 31; Greek]*

Further evidence of such a phenomenon was seen in Andrew's *[Andrew, GP, age early 40s; Greek]* enjoyment in getting the medical business out of the way so that he could talk with his patient, and, in a striking example, in Theodore's *[Theodore, GP, age 63; Greek]* reminiscing about his former patients at their grave-sites. Margarita *[Margarita, GP, age 33; Greek]* offered a similar style of response when asked of what rewards the process of care offered:

> **MARGARITA** I think it's the ... life experience for me. It's life experience. ... It's umm, going into something a little more deeper and, being a part of a process and ... you know, it makes me sort of think about life in general when ... I'm involved with these sort of things. ... And, ... it makes me sort of walk away and think, "Well", you know, "like it's interesting how life sort of blossoms and ... comes to an end at some stage", and I, I, I think, for me it's that sort of life experience.   *[Margarita, GP, age 33; Greek]*

Such positive experiences, however, seemed paradoxical because they could only be fully realised in circumstances where the doctor was also maximally committed to dealing with the negative and disturbing aspects of the illness:

> **ANDREW** ... it will be calls after hours, after you finish surgery, in the middle of the night, early in the morning. Again I do those because I have to do them because they must be done. ... I mean, if you've decided to treat someone because they're dying then you've got to do, ... do the whole works, you can't just do half of it.   *[Andrew, GP, age early 40s; Greek]*

And again:

> **ANDREW** ... I think it's [i.e. the reward is] the motivation that you're caring and concerned for the, for your patients, for the person that's going through this particular suffering and ... , who really is as I see it probably feeling very, very alone in the world and very, very frightened ... and I think ... I don't think there could be anything more frightening than that, ... than to feel alone. ... Even when you are surrounded by your family and what ever, but also people do abandon you at this time. So I guess I feel very committed to people like this because they're going through a very difficult predicament.
>
> *[Andrew, GP, age early 40s; Greek]*

Cancer as struggle

'Cancer as struggle' differed slightly from the concept of cancer as loss. Whereas the latter was universal, the struggle against it varied between individuals as well as within the individual themselves according to the stage of the illness and the type of cancer present. That struggle itself (or lack of it) formed the central theme in some of the interviews.

Struggle could have varying aims, such as cure, maintenance of stability, or the exercise of some degree of *control* over aspects of management. Sometimes struggle constituted an effort to support others in dealing with the illness, which in turn affected the person themselves in terms of their own coping. An example of this was given by Monica *[Monica, age 48 with breast cancer; Alan, age late 50s—husband; Anglo-Celtic]*, who lost her hair because of chemotherapy but helped her daughter to *confront* the loss by having confronted it herself:

> **MONICA** ... as my hair started to grow, it was tiny, tiny short but I'd been ... to the hairdresser and he used the number two razor all over ... and we put a rinse in because it comes back white ... and we put a rinse in to my normal colour so that it looked as if there was more there. And then around [the] house I'd just stopped wearing hats. It was September—October, it was getting warm. And one night ... I walked into the kitchen and April's saying, ... "Go out, Byron's here". ... And I said, "No". ... I walked into the kitchen. I was determined not to run and put the hat on because I ... thought at this point April had to confront it. ... And it was at home at night, she wasn't going out—we could talk it out if we had to. ... And Byron took one look at me and said, "Oh, you can come to army with me if you like!" [both laugh]. And April relaxed. It was just lovely. ... It was the perfect comment. ... And she's, she's coped with that much

better this time, but this time, I guess 'cause I was a lot sicker … she doesn't say much at all now.

[Monica, age 48 with breast cancer; Alan, age late 50s—husband; Anglo-Celtic]

Struggle, however, also had to have some element of realism in order to be most effective and to avoid degenerating into denial. Whereas Panteleimon's *[Panteleimon, age 62 with lung cancer; Mary, age 63—wife; Greek]* initial lack of struggle was disproportionate in relation to his condition (see above, p. 29), the opposite scenario could also be quite difficult to cope with. Such a scenario was seen with George *[George, age mid-50s with lung cancer; Katerina, age ?—wife; Greek]*, who hoped to live on to see his children more established, and also to become a grandfather, despite having end-stage metastatic lung cancer. This caused concern and sadness for his wife, who knew that death was imminent:

FIELD NOTES He still has hopes of getting well, and she does not quash these, but realises that there will come a time when he will not be able to say the things that he wants to say, and I presumed that Katerina meant that he would not get a chance to say goodbye. This seems a dilemma for her.

[George, age mid-50s with lung cancer; Katerina, age ?—wife; Greek]

Despite the usually poor prognosis in cancer, medical struggle against the illness was not always negative, depressing or engaged without enthusiasm. For example, as shown above under 'Cancer as gain', the struggle against cancer was at times personally and spiritually rewarding. The medical struggle could also be scientifically interesting and rewarding. Jane's *[Jane, English, age 61 with mycosis fungoides; John, German, age 70—husband]* relationship with her dermatologist, for example, in many ways hinged on the scientific interest that her rare condition and her unexpectedly prolonged survival aroused in him. The dermatologist's main interest in Jane's condition itself, rather than in her as a person, did not bother Jane, but rather made her feel secure:

JANE Well, I don't think it [i.e. the doctor's interest] was really personal, I don't think it was because he liked me; … it was his curiosity, his, his desire for knowledge of the complaint. … And … the different aspects of it, and how it … especially in me, … seeing it was a bit … variant, I obviously was reacting differently to every body else. … That unsettled him, he wanted, he wanted answers … He's very good and … he doesn't waste time. He's very, very busy and his time is very precious.

[Jane, English, age 61 with mycosis fungoides; John, German, age 70—husband]

The notion of a positive, willing medical struggle (a 'challenge') was also seen in the observations of Delvecchio-Good, Good, Schaffer & Lind (1990), who noted that 'confronting the biological frontiers of disease and the commitment to altering those frontiers' motivated many American oncologists. A similar sense of challenge was also seen with the GP informants but was focused more at the level of symptom control and emotional comfort, rather than on contributing new biomedical knowledge to medicine about the particular cancer type.

Cancer as self

Although cancer was generally seen as 'non-self', as something foreign or alien, circumstances sometimes linked it closely to the notion of 'self'. Cancer could therefore, simultaneously and paradoxically, be 'self' and 'non-self', as also observed by Gordon (1990).

Causal behaviour, such as cigarette smoking and lung cancer (seen with Panteleimon [*Panteleimon, age 62 with lung cancer; Mary, age 63—wife; Greek]*), advanced cervical cancer after never having had a Papanicolaou smear test (seen with Barbara [*Barbara, age 48 with cervical cancer; Dimitri, age 53—husband; Greek]*), or diagnosis of advanced disease after delays in attending to physical symptoms (seen with Clare [*Clare, age 65 with stomach cancer; Michael, age 67—husband; Anglo-Celtic]*) had the potential to morally link and identify the patient with their illness. The illness itself often either consciously or sub-consciously invoked consideration of the causal behaviour, usually by persons other than the patient.

Sometimes, without implying a direct, conscious and causal link between a specific behaviour and illness, the illness could reflect the individual personality and constitutional make-up of the patient on a more general level. Sontag (1978), for example, reflecting on the romantic associations of tuberculosis, noted it to be an illness of delicate, expressive and creative persons. Cancer, however, is an illness with a more sinister reputation. If 'feelings about evil are projected onto a disease' and that 'the disease (so enriched with meanings) is projected onto the world' (Sontag, 1978: 58), then by association those feelings are also reflected back upon the patient themselves. Cancer could therefore potentially imply a stifled, repressed or unhealthy manner of living, or a poor emotional or physical constitution. The disease thus came to represent the moral 'failure' of the patient for not avoiding it. The commentary of Margarita [*Margarita, GP, age 33; Greek]*, a GP who rigidly emphasised a healthy diet, 'stress management', and 'relaxation techniques' as keys to good health, illustrated such feeling:

MARGARITA They're [i.e. Greeks] very much … , "I want …a drug", sort of thing, "I want tablet", whatever, and when you talk to them … , "Look, if you give up smoking, … you give up coffee, you eat more fruit and vegetables, your blood pressure will come down", things like that. What I find, they don't do that, but they're prepared to take the tablets. … They're very religious with the tablets. … That … very, very obstinate [approach], so, that's the other fact that I find with … Greek(s) … it could be with other cultures but, … a *lot* [emphasised] of the patients that I see here … [are] very highly motivated. … Very highly motivated patients. So, it could, I'm not sure what it is. So I think they [the Greeks] need more training in that way. *[Margarita, GP, age 33; Greek]*

The notion of cancer as 'self' was sometimes extended or conferred to *healthy* persons because of their intimate links to the patient. In those circumstances, the illness devastated the carer as much as it did the patient. Cancer could therefore become a *family* entity rather than an entity of the patient alone:

PETER … [I'm] melancholic all the time, always … with agony, with … how can one say it, … what will happen? Maybe she will leave us, she will be finished. Then, our life is useless for us. … We … are always idle, in great agony … [about] what will happen, how she will progress. … She notices weakness and I am sad all the time. … I am always, always thinking [about this]. … Might something happen to her? From there on, I am also finished. What will I do by myself? …
INTERVIEWER You have the family, though …
PETER Well, I have the family, but the companion is the companion.
[Maria, age 69 with breast cancer; Peter, age 74—husband; Greek]

Cancer as 'self' could also be more solidly built into one's physical make-up. One striking example related to the thoughts of a young man who had many relatives affected by cancer, including his father, Simon *[Simon, age 64 with lymphoma; Cynthia, age 52—wife; Anglo-Celtic]*. Such a family history meant that his own body, according to its genetic structure, was almost predestined to developing the disease, thereby in essence linking his notion of 'self' to the disease in a powerful way:

CYNTHIA … Peter … is concerned to the point 'will it come out on him?'. … Will he get it [i.e. cancer]? … He said, "With the family history", … he said, "what hope have I got?"
[Simon, age 64 with lymphoma; Cynthia, age 52—wife; Anglo-Celtic]

In a similar but perhaps less binding way, cancer could also be viewed as 'self' by persons around the patient, because it was *possible* that they or others close to them might in future also suffer from it. As observed by Dozor & Addison (1992), such personal discomfort produced by the lack of immunity over death was a considerable stressor for doctors:

FRANK ... as an emotional experience it [i.e. death] can be a, a humbling experience ... and yet it's, I think, ... a, a fundamental component of general practice that we should get involved in, even if it involves overcoming ... our own inadequacies, I suppose, about death and, and the remaining aspects.

[Frank, GP, age early 30s; Anglo-Celtic]

Other informants related the process of cancer to 'self' by their conception of death as a natural process. The cancer they lived with and dealt with was a part of life, and not something totally foreign. Overall satisfaction with life and a minimisation of loss were, however, important determinants in the prominence of such thinking:

CHARLES ... well, when I look around and see little kids with it [i.e. cancer] I think, you know, what the hell should I worry about?, you know. ... I've had a good life and I've, I've had a terrific life.

[Charles, age 72 with prostate cancer; Amanda, age 72—wife; Anglo-Celtic]

Charmaz (1983) discussed the impact of chronic illness upon the self but referred only to *losses* of roles and *negative, restrictive* changes in self concept. She stated that 'chronically ill persons frequently experience a crumbling away of their former self-images *without* simultaneous development of equally valid new ones. ... Over time, accumulated loss of formerly sustaining self-images *without new ones* results in a diminished self-concept' (Charmaz, 1983: 168; emphasis added secondarily). However, the examples presented here illustrate that changes in self-concept are not always negative and destructive. The illness simultaneously gave the individual (patient, carer or GP) new insights into their own mortality and personal vulnerability, and therefore a *greater*, albeit *different*, insight of their own self. That was further reinforced through the various *gains* that were also possible through the illness. Charmaz (1983: 191) yielded to this point at the very end of her paper by briefly mentioning, as an exception, 'those who had improved and no longer suffered as greatly as they had in the past. These individuals were more likely to see their earlier suffering as a path to knowledge and self-discovery'. However, based on the evidence provided here, even this concession seemed under-emphasised. The findings here suggest that gains through illness and in positive contributions to the self-concept were not uncommon, and further, that they were possible even for patients who were still *actively suffering*. While the presence of such gains did not *negate* the anguish caused by cancer-related loss, they could and did alter how such losses were perceived.

The heightened awareness of self caused by cancer was not only dependent on the internal, emotional reaction towards the illness, but also upon the individual's outward responses towards the illness situation. These were also important contributors towards the revelation of the 'true' or the 'real' self, as implied by the Greek proverb that 'the skill of the captain is only manifest on rough seas'. In that light, social expectations to fight cancer, so popular in American culture (Delvecchio-Good et al., 1990; Saillant, 1990), either commend the patient or alternatively condemn them if they do not put up a 'good' or a 'brave' fight.

Further, the style of coping and sense of self in an individual also influenced and shaped the coping and self-concept of others around them. This in turn was dynamically fed back to the person and further moulded their own self-perceptions and methods of coping. The self-concept was thus shaped through complex interactions with others. Consider, for example, the situation of Clare *[Clare, age 65 with stomach cancer; Michael, age 67—husband; Anglo-Celtic]*, who accepted her illness and was a major source of support in helping her husband to cope with it. Her strength, in fact, depended in part upon his:

> **MICHAEL** ... I put my arms around her and I ... I'd sort of blubber a bit. She'd say, "Now, come on, how do you expect me to carry on?" [becomes very emotional at this point, and eyes watering].
>
> *[Clare, age 65 with stomach cancer; Michael, age 67—husband; Anglo-Celtic]*

Cancer as uncertain or unknown

The lack of knowledge about the cause of many types of cancer made it a mysterious illness, and such mystery could heighten the inherent fear of it (Sontag, 1978). Further uncertainty about cancer after it was diagnosed occurred at two levels.

First, there was uncertainty in families and doctors alike about the future clinical progress of the disease. Even when the natural history of the disease was well understood, the element of unpredictability always remained. Precise details of temporal progression, symptom magnitude, functional effects, responses to treatment, and potential complications remained unpredictable. Additionally, even when medical predictions about illness events were accurate, such predictions could not convey what it would be like to actually *experience them*—that remained completely unknown until the time itself came (Kellehear, 1990). Such uncertainty often placed patient and family in a no-win situation regarding knowledge of the condition, because both the presence of knowledge or the lack of it could be anxiety provoking. Panteleimon's *[Panteleimon, age 62 with lung cancer; Mary, age 63—wife; Greek]* withdrawal into himself on learning of the diagnosis probably reflected elements of such anxiety that related to the uncertainty of future experiences. Such was also the case with Paraskevi *[Paraskevi, age 48 with cervical cancer; Mark, age 23—son; Greek]*:

FIELD NOTES Mark accompanied me barefoot to my car on my way out. He told me that Paraskevi was not fully aware of the extent of the illness. Apparently the cancer has gone "everywhere", to bones, to many other sites. Paraskevi recently had problems with the left kidney, presumably obstructive difficulties, but the family told her that she was being treated for an infection. Mark feels that Paraskevi may lose hope if fully aware, as on initial diagnosis, she, who had been previously reasonably active, suddenly became bed-ridden. ...

[Paraskevi, age 48 with cervical cancer; Mark, age 23—son; Greek]

Second, there was uncertainty related to the understanding of what cancer actually *was*, in a more specific manner than its metaphorical conception of being foreign and nasty. Lay descriptions of the pathophysiology of cancer had different levels of emphasis. For example:

INTERVIEWER ... What do you understand ... about what sort of a sickness it is? How does this sickness work? ...
PANTELEIMON Eh, you will notice that your nerves are paralysed. You notice that your body becomes paralysed. ... You don't have strength. ... You don't have any appetite. ... Ah, certainly you notice that you are not progressing well. ...
INTERVIEWER ... Your feelings about the cancer that ... it is a bad illness, how did you develop these? Why did you think that it was a bad illness?
PANTELEIMON Eh, given that you hear that this certain [person] died. "What did he have?" "Ah, cancer.'

[Panteleimon, age 62 with lung cancer; Mary, age 63—wife; Greek]

Despite the fact that Panteleimon *[Panteleimon, age 62 with lung cancer; Mary, age 63—wife; Greek]* had suffered from bowel cancer some ten years earlier, and had been cured by a colectomy, his view of cancer was framed largely in terms of its effects upon the body, especially its ability to generate weakness and pain. The ability to delineate and appreciate the illness according to its *pathology* (for example type, site, extent, potential for progress or cure), in addition to its symptom profile, seemed greater among Anglo-Celtic informants and among the more educated informants. That could either facilitate or hinder the appreciation of the varying aims of medical therapy. Examples were seen in circumstances where therapy aimed to reduce disease burden but produced side-effects. Such therapy might not be as appreciated if the patient's main focus was upon their *symptomatic* well-being.

In some cases, understanding of cancer went beyond the physical manifestations by attempts to link them to events at the cellular level:

INTERVIEWER ... What do you think is happening with your skin? ...

JANE Well as far as I know it's in the ah red blood cells. And it causes the white blood cells, the white corpuscles, to accelerate so my white blood count is way higher than my red. ... And it erupts through the skin in the form of sores, lesions, papules, papulars, whatever you call them.

[Jane, English, age 61 with mycosis fungoides; John, German, age 70—husband]

Although such understanding was not always scientifically accurate, as in Jane's case above, it was generally linked to a greater awareness of the *purpose* and *scope* of treatment. Treatments could therefore be recounted and differentiated according to their specific purpose. Such understanding alone often conferred some perceived *control* over the situation (although as stated, poor perceived control, fear and other factors could limit information-seeking about the illness).

As the biomedical understanding of cancer increased, medical interventions were also more fully appreciated and *psychologically integrated* into the illness trajectory. That could be both positive and negative. For example, Monica *[Monica, age 48 with breast cancer; Alan, age late 50s—husband; Anglo-Celtic]*, with her detailed understanding of the pathophysiology of her inflammatory breast cancer, knew that the squeezing of her breast by an early mammogram had enhanced the risk of tumour cells dislodging and metastasising. However, in general, her detailed knowledge of the illness and its treatment benefited her. Names of chemotherapy drugs, details of histopathology reports, statistical prognosis, different management options, and many other details were well known—this conferred a sense of control that enabled her to remain involved with her treatment and progress.

In the final analysis, enhancing the biomedical understanding of patients and families (without disregarding or trivialising other ways of understanding cancer) was a delicate process. Sometimes it imparted a sense of *meaning* and *control* in treatment, but sometimes too much knowledge was a negative factor that was undesirable and destructive, engendering excessive fear and gloom.

Cancer as a test

Cancer often evoked speculation and comment about God. Some informants, such as Charles *[Charles, age 72 with prostate cancer; Amanda, age 72—wife; Anglo-Celtic]* did not believe in God's existence because they felt that God would not test persons with cancer. Many religious families, however, saw cancer as an illness allowed by God. Major events in the illness, often the diagnosis, were frequently recalled in relation to their temporal proximity to important Christian periods, such as Lent, Easter, Christmas, or the Dormition of the Virgin Mary (as seen in *[Maria, age 69 with breast cancer; Peter, age 74—husband; Greek]*, *[George, age mid-50s with lung cancer; Katerina, age ?—wife; Greek]*, *[Panteleimon, age 62 with lung cancer; Mary, age 63—wife; Greek]*, and *[Simon, age 64 with lymphoma; Cynthia, age 52—wife; Anglo-Celtic]*). Holy icons were seen in bedrooms, and the Cross was often worn visibly around the neck. Their faith that God would be with them, no matter what the outcome, assisted such families in their overall coping:

> **FIELD NOTES** ... She [Aristotle's wife] asked why God had allowed him to come down with this illness. She crossed herself in the Orthodox Christian manner and accepted his plight as God's will.
>
> *[Aristotle, age 79 with prostate cancer; Paula, age ?—daughter; Greek]*

> **FIELD NOTES** Katerina seemed religious and made references to things being in God's hands. ...
>
> *[George, age mid-50s with lung cancer; Katerina, age ?—wife; Greek]*

> **MARY** ... like us, who leave it to rest upon God, they [i.e. the doctors] do the same.
>
> *[Panteleimon, age 62 with lung cancer; Mary, age 63—wife; Greek]*

CYNTHIA I do a *lot* [emphasised] of talking to God. It's not just of a night time, but during the day, it's any time.

[Simon, age 64 with lymphoma; Cynthia, age 52—wife; Anglo-Celtic]

Whether they were religious or not, all GPs acknowledged the importance of religion to families and all encouraged this if families had embraced it. GPs also actively used religion to help patients to come to an acceptance of their situation:

INTERVIEWER So if they'll say to you, you know, "I haven't got long doc", or whatever ...?
THEODORE Oŋly God knows. [spoken in Greek]

[Theodore, GP, age 63; Greek]

And again:

BYRON ... from a Christian perspective I think I don't ... fear death and ah I like to ...impart that to patients. ... I ... hate ... patients being told, "Oh, You've got ah two weeks to live", or something like this. I'm always pretty positive ..., "Don't give up, ... you've got plenty of enjoy. You've enjoyed having your aunt come in yesterday to see you ... and ... there's plenty more to live for, and ... none of us ever know when we're going to die and ...". ... There's a lot of positive reassuring that usually you can give them along those lines. ... And that, "Whether you're here or whether you're there, you know, God will look after you", and ... this sort of [thing], ... being positive. ... "It's not [as though] you go into some cold, dreary, unfeeling place when you do die ... ." But ... often I suppose [it's] more saying, "Well, it's warm and comfortable here, you've got a roof over your head and ... you've got a chance to put your affairs in order and get it right with the family, and ... it's much better than motor car accidents and being killed on the road or having a heart attack in bed. There's a lot that's ... OK about ... terminal illness that's ah protracted a little bit, ... as long as we can give you pain relief ... aɴd make you feel comfortable."

[Byron, GP, age 57; Anglo-Celtic]

Cancer, however, was also a test in non–spiritual terms. It was a test in coping with adversity and massive change. It was therefore also a test of self and self-control:

MARIA ... The psychological rest is—today the friend coming over, tomorrow the compatriot, tomorrow the brother, I don't know how, because the life [that I now lead] is closed, it is not free. ... And slowly—slowly one becomes used to this sort of life. ... The beginnings have their own difficulty, because ... you are in pain, that you can't move ... Well, will you then start to say, "I'm in pain, I will die? O, ... save me my child, save me? My daughter, save me?" But we understand ... what ... [the problem] is; we try [to alleviate it]; ... beyond that ... they can't [cure it].

[Maria, age 69 with breast cancer; Peter, age 74—husband; Greek]

The ramifications of such self-control were important in helping others to cope, as seen with Clare's support of Michael:

MICHAEL ... I saw the doctor come out ... [and] then she [i.e. Clare] come out, ... "Well", she said, "It's the worst." I said, "Yes." She said, "I've got cancer." You know, I said to her, "Oh... that's terrible. ... I'm amazed at the way that you're taking it," you know, which I was. ... And so she said, ... "Don't worry, ... I asked the doctor and ... she was saying yes, with this type of cancer ... there's things can be done with it, ... its not the finish, you know". ...

[Clare, age 65 with stomach cancer; Michael, age 67—husband; Anglo-Celtic]

Cancer as a determined outcome

Distinct from the notion of accepting cancer as a part of life, the view of cancer was sometimes most emphasised and characterised by a *causative* or *determinant* element. Beliefs about cancer causation took on varying levels of emphasis and fell into several categories. Often there was no clear postulate from the family as to why the cancer had occurred, and in those cases the 'how' (that is, the aetiology) was not a prominent theme. It was uncertain, a *chance* occurrence. Others, particularly the more religious and well adjusted, saw the occurrence of cancer as *destiny*. Still others emphasised *personal habits, family history, work* or *environment* factors as causative issues. No striking cultural differences were noted in these respects.

Habit-related factors on the part of the patient, were usually more strongly emphasised by the relatives rather than the patient. Of the GPs, Margarita's *[Margarita, GP, age 33; Greek]* narrative particularly emphasised patients' general 'failings' in their general lifestyle habits, reflecting her own strong views on those issues. Habit-related causative factors did not so centrally occupy the narratives of the other GPs.

Work and *environment* factors, outside immediate personal control, tended to be emphasised more by the patients themselves, as well as their carers. With some Greek families, the industrial workplace took on particular prominence:

INTERVIEWER ... Do you have any idea about ... why you have become ill with ... cancer? ...

PANTELEIMON What idea can one put up first? ... There at the foundry where I worked ... the metal was melting, [and] we ... we divided it amongst the moulds. ... When you poured the metal ... there [was] a, a smoke. ... You take the steel alight, half heated up, so as to throw it to the side. ... All of the dust was given off. ... Where were all of these going? ... [implying that his body absorbed the fumes and dust]. ... Every night, whether it was raining or snowing, you had to have a bath [before leaving work], because [otherwise] you could not get dressed. ... The overalls from the morning up until night-time were soaked ... in sweat. ... Well then, what do you expect from this body?

[Panteleimon, age 62 with lung cancer; Mary, age 63—wife; Greek]

Although Mary, Panteleimon's wife, felt that his smoking was heavily implicated in causing the lung cancer, she agreed with him on the foundry issue:

MARY ... I think that it might have played a role—the dust. The pillowcases ... were permeated [with the smell] ... [i.e. the smell of metal was imparted to them by Panteleimon's head]. ... Even if he did wash, there was so much that his body went through, even the sweat soaked the bedsheets. ... Ah, from, from this steel ... the sweat ... where the ... the permeated smell stayed in it and it couldn't be cleaned away. *[Panteleimon, age 62 with lung cancer; Mary, age 63—wife; Greek]*

More general stressors, such as the difficult childhood mentioned by Jane *[Jane, English, age 61 with mycosis fungoides; John, German, age 70— husband]*, were also suspected to have played a causative role in the development of cancer.

The cancer world of the clinician

The cancer world of the clinician was closely tied to their professional role as a healer. Although immersed in the emotion-laden world of patients and families through their intimate contact with them, it was the doctor's *therapeutic role* that ultimately defined their presence and purpose in the relationship.

The GP informants demonstrated six distinct ways of understanding the therapeutic approach towards cancer, each of which had important implications for the doctor–patient relationship. These categories of thinking are summarised in Box 1.2.

BOX 1.2 Emphasis placed on cancer by GPs

The 'epidemiological' emphasis	The 'disease-burden' emphasis
The 'functional' emphasis	The 'intuitive' emphasis
The 'chronicity' emphasis	The 'partnership' emphasis.

Before a formal analysis of each of these emphases, their essence will be briefly sketched in a hypothetical scenario of a 65-year-old man with a 4-millimetre-thick malignant melanoma on the left cheek and no detectable metastases.

A malignant melanoma of 4 millimetres thickness has a poor long-term prognosis (Kumar & Clark, 1994). An *'epidemiological' emphasis* in care sees all management decisions overshadowed by the poor long-term survival statistics. The *'disease-burden' emphasis* adopts a different view by being satisfied that the patient can be rendered 'macroscopically cancer-free' by widely excising the lesion. If rib and spine metastases appear, the disease-burden can no longer be removed. The patient, however, might respond to palliative radiotherapy and be rendered pain-free and able to walk. The doctor oriented around the *'functional' emphasis* is highly satisfied with this. Towards the latter stages of illness, however, functional and symptomatic decline may eventuate, and death is not far away—or is it? The *'intuitive' emphasis* sees the human hope of the GP rise above seemingly insurmountable decline. Could the patient be that 'one in a million' person who defies the odds?

Other GPs emphasised the *chronicity* of cancer and its management, irrespective of its prognosis, extent, functional consequences, or any personal intuitions they held about it. This made cancer akin to other chronic illnesses such as osteoarthritis or emphysema, whose continuation and progression is expected, anticipated and *actively* engaged. Still other GPs emphasised *partnership* with the patient and family above all else in the palliative care process. In its absence, such GPs would be unsatisfied with the process of care even if symptom control and other aspects of management had proceeded smoothly.

This prelude has also hinted that these therapeutic emphases were *not static over time*. As the illness progressed, the orientation of management had to be continually refined, shifting, for example, from hopes of initial cure, to hopes of disease control, to hopes of symptom control. Disease progress thus dictated the *practical* realities of management. In our hypothetical case, a GP might have progressed from an initially epidemiological orientation, to that of a disease-burden orientation, to that of a functional orientation as illness progression forced hopes further from the ideal (that is, cure) and closer towards the practical (that is, symptomatic and functional control). However, it was also plausible that the epidemiologically oriented GP might have been *unable* to encompass other modes of thinking about the illness. Although 'mechanically' supporting and caring for the patient as they deteriorated, the predominating medical attitude might therefore remain focused on ultimate loss and be unable to appreciate functional or other symptomatic gains. Obviously, this could hold major repercussions on the attitudes and coping of patient and family. The completely opposite scenario (that is, excessive GP hope in obviously end-stage illness) could also do the same.

Additionally, the systems of thinking about cancer management were *not mutually exclusive*, and could coexist in varying combinations. The intuitive component for either good or poor progress, for example, could respectively coexist with firm epidemiological evidence suggesting the opposite. Likewise, a focus on doctor–patient partnership or illness chronicity could coexist with functional, disease-burden or epidemiological emphases. The *individually* elaborated systems of thinking about the palliative care tasks which follow must therefore be read with these points in mind.

The 'epidemiological' emphasis

This emphasis was shaped by pre-existing medical knowledge about the natural history of the particular cancer type. Although function was an important criterion of illness status, attention was more centrally focused on the likelihood of long-term survival, irrespective of the patient's current physical condition. All medical actions were thus psychologically grounded on anticipated outcomes according to epidemiological knowledge of the illness.

By nature of their cure-oriented training, all GPs related to this framework. By moulding the context of the GP's overall approach to care, the expected progression of illness therefore shaped the nature and expression of the patient-centred approach itself. Such a shaping was often subtle, but could nonetheless generate a degree of reservation that affected even the most well-meaning patient-centred approaches. An example was found in comments about cancer patients in remission but who were likely to relapse:

ANDREW ... And ... they'll finish their radiotherapy and they'll come back from the specialist and they'll say, you know, "The specialist said to me that he's really pleased with me, he said that I've done well, that we've got this under control and I've had all these scans and ... they haven't found any tumour at all, there's no secondaries in the bone, in the liver and the blood tests are okay; isn't that great?" And you think, "Yeah, that is great", you know, and you feel really good for them but you know deep down ... in a few months it's not really going to be great and you will be back here and you're going to say to me, "How come?" ... So how do we address that? What do we say to them? I mean, do we shatter their hopes?

[Andrew, GP, age early 40s; Greek]

Sometimes, however, doctors' discomfort with poor prognosis was strong enough to influence the patient–centred approach more heavily. Those circumstances powerfully shaped how families felt about and understood the illness. Such an instance was described by an informant who had witnessed the disclosure of bowel cancer to a hospital patient by a resident doctor:

CYNTHIA ... this gentleman had been losing some weight. ... And the chap in the next cubicle area ... he was ... sitting in the chair ... and ah this young lady, a young doctor just walked in. She was just looking all around, just looked all around the room. ... And she said to him ... , "I have some news to tell you". She said, "You have got bowel cancer". [pause] It's just ... it was the way she said it. ... She just said ... , "I'll be around after to speak to you". ... And just left it at that. And of course the gentleman just broke down.

[Simon, age 64 with lymphoma; Cynthia, age 52—wife; Anglo-Celtic]

The silence, body language and lack of elaboration by the hospital doctor plainly conveyed an anticipated poor outlook to the patient. Work-related pressures could also enhance the emphasis of the epidemiological approach. Groopman (1987), for instance, in an extreme example, described how sleep deprivation in American interns and resident doctors made them bitterly *resent* treating persons with an irretrievably poor prognosis. Such extremes in working conditions, however, were not seen in GP informants to this study.

Many patients and families, especially if the patient was symptomatically well, were made uncomfortable by negative medical orientations that were conveyed either consciously or unconsciously by health personnel. Such discomfort did not equate to denial, but rather to expectations that the 'truth' should be tempered or balanced with information about positive aspects in treatment or prognosis. That psychological need was especially prominent in Greek patients and carers, but was also seen with Anglo-Celtic informants:

> **INTERVIEWER** How was the disclosure made?
> **MONICA** It was, "Oh, that's an inflammatory cancer. I want a mammogram". ... I guess at that stage I just wanted something to happen quickly. ... Alan and I are both pretty straight from the shoulder. ... I'd like it ... to be straight, open and honest ... but ... there was *no softening afterwards* [emphasis added, not actual] ...
>
> *[Monica, age 48 with breast cancer; Alan, age late 50s—husband; Anglo-Celtic]*

Unlike the theorising of Kubler-Ross (1969), which used the word 'denial' to describe patterns of early reactions to a terminal illness, this phenomenon seemed more like a tendency towards *normalisation,* and was active *even in advanced stages of illness,* as seen with Barbara, whose advanced cervical cancer caused gross peripheral oedema that confined her to bed or a chair for most of the day:

> **INTERVIEWER** ... You told me that you had done a few dishes today in the morning.
> **BARBARA** Yes, yes, ... I washed the dishes a little ... and yesterday I washed the dishes. ... I started bit by bit to do a certain small chore so that I might recover from the numbness that I get from [sitting in] the chair.
>
> *[Barbara, age 48 with cervical cancer; Dimitri, age 53—husband; Greek]*

It seemed then that the epidemiological emphasis of doctors was not incompatible with patients and families in terms of the grimness of its message, but rather in terms of how that message was delivered and acted upon by the medical profession.

The 'disease-burden' emphasis

This emphasis in management shifted the ultimate focus of care away from the distant future (where the epidemiological approach was focused) towards the more immediate future. The outlook took a shorter-term view of illness status, and as such it centred not so much on known epidemiology but rather on diagnosis of disease burden or disease dissemination or progression. Even though a patient might be *functionally* well, it was recurrence, persistent high disease burden, or progression of cancer that dulled the hope of ongoing survival and shaped feelings about the scope and purpose of ongoing care. More distant, potential outcomes played a less central role in shaping the current approach.

There were various markers that defined the notion of disease burden, ranging from clinically detectable disease extent, site of disease, cell counts, histological tumour type, status of tumour markers and other biochemical changes, and radiologically detectable extent of disease.

The disease-burden classification was especially emphasised where the tumour was no longer detectable in the body after treatment, or if the overall tumour burden was small. There, human hope among patient, family and doctor could prevail over unfavourable epidemiological predictions. Simon *[Simon, age 64 with lymphoma; Cynthia, age 52—wife; Anglo-Celtic]*, for example, had a residual nodule of lymphoma in his skin at the elbow following chemotherapy, but was not too concerned because it was small, external and visible; the potentially more dangerous and unknown internal lesions had been rendered undetectable by treatment.

Recurrent cycles of relapse, treatment and subsequent remission could, however, exact an emotional toll that somewhat dimmed the hope of a prolonged survival even with minimal or no disease burden:

CYNTHIA I mean it looks like it's going to be an ongoing thing. ... In the early stages you could say, "Yes, you've got rid of it and that's the finish of it", ... but ... this has gone on nearly seven years now. And ... you just don't know when they're [i.e. the lymphoma deposits] gonna appear. ... And the thing is they appear back in the same spots as where they started ... I used to write it down in the diary, the dates and all that. I don't do that now. I used to do that 'cause Simon would like to refer back ... to ... , you know, how many months that broke out and all the rest of it. Well he did that for a few years but we ... I don't do that now ... And ... you just don't know when they're gonna break out and ... when he finds them you think, "Oh, not again".

[Simon, age 64 with lymphoma; Cynthia, age 52—wife; Anglo-Celtic]

If used as a prognostic guide in the context of relatively stable, non-advanced illness that was amenable to treatment, the disease-burden emphasis of the doctor could aid family and patient coping even if the cancer was incurable. The optimistic approach by many specialists that was noted above by Andrew *[Andrew, GP, age early 40s; Greek]* might have represented such an attempt, although it trod the perilous line between generating *unrealistic* optimism as opposed to *realistic* optimism:

ANDREW ... I think what you have to address are different concerns like ... treatment, side effects of treatment, prospects of cure, prospects of just control, what are we doing, I mean what's the point of all of this, ... "Why should I be making myself so sick of all this therapy if I'm going to die anyway?", ... those sorts of questions need to be addressed. [These] questions are very poorly addressed by the specialties because they're just, patients are just going there, they're having their treatment. You know, "We're are going to cure you, we're going to fix you, we're going to beat it", you know.

[Andrew, GP, age early 40s; Greek]

However, even those doctors, patients and carers who were 'realistic' and were aware of an ultimately poor prognosis would not fully yield to the illness psychologically until it showed evidence of significant progression. Again, this was because the time–frame of orientation was in the present and near future, rather than the distant future.

The 'functional' emphasis

Some GPs were primarily oriented towards the functional status of their patients, *irrespective* of either epidemiological outlooks or disease burden status. Many patients with unfavourable illness were functionally stable. Palliative care in such a framework began when function and stability were being lost:

INTERVIEWER ... On what sort of criteria do, do we usually make this decision that someone is *palliative*? [word emphasised] ...

ANDREW ... It's not an easy one to answer because the palliative [state] starts at different stages for different people for different problems I think. ... I don't think it starts necessarily with the diagnosis, ... although, [pause] for me as a doctor when you get the diagnosis you know more or less what the ... what the long-term thing is going to be. ... What you don't know is, [pause] ... Let me phrase that a little bit differently. ... There's a stage between the diagnosis and the palliative state. For me the palliative state is when somebody ... is starting on the decline. ... When everything that could possibly be done to try and keep this tumour at bay, to keep it under control, has been done and [it] is now out of control. ... And you know that from now on it is down hill. ... That there, for me, that's the palliative state. Now the state from diagnosis to the palliative state can be short, can be long. ... And what happens in that period is varied quite considerably.

[Andrew, GP, age early 40s; Greek]

GPs with such a definition of palliative care were certainly aware of the ultimate reality of decline and often did not ignore or conceal it, but they appreciated the relative wellness of their patients *now*, and how such wellness enabled these patients to live peacefully and meaningfully. Table 1.1 summarises how this outlook compares to the epidemiological and disease-burden approaches by showing where projected outlooks are grounded in terms of time. Table 1.2 furthers this notion by comparing functional versus epidemiological modes of response across different scenarios.

TABLE 1.1 Time-orientations of different palliative care approaches

APPROACH	CONTEXT
Functional	'now'
Disease-burden	'immediate future'
Epidemiological	'distant future'

TABLE 1.2 *Functional* versus **epidemiological** modes of medical response

	Treatment offers potential for long-term survival ± cure	Treatment cannot offer long-term survival
Patient symptomatically well	*Medical confidence* **Medical confidence**	*Medical contentment* **Medical condolence**
Patient symptomatically unwell	*Medical concern* **Medical reassurance**	*Medical palliation* **Medical helplessness**

In the functional sense, palliative care was more or less equivalent to 'terminal care', or care of the incapacitated patient near the end-stage of their illness. Such a view of palliative care could be labelled by the epidemiologically minded as misleading and inaccurate. However, its orientation was humane because of its efforts to maximise the notion of normality.

Most patients and families assessed the progress and ultimate prognosis of their condition based on function, even when, according to the disease-burden and epidemiological emphases, prognosis was not optimistic:

FIELD NOTES Monica's ... condition had significantly improved to the point where she was now getting on with things, including "learning to walk again". She noted that although she probably still has a bit more "chemo" to go through, she is getting on with things and moving ahead.

[*Monica, age 48 with breast cancer; Alan, age late 50s—husband; Anglo-Celtic*]

The *visual appearance* of the patient was incorporated into the notion of function, particularly by people other than the patient, who used it to gauge functional capacity and well-being (recall Monica's *[Monica, age 48 with breast cancer; Alan, age late 50s—husband; Anglo-Celtic]* hair loss from chemotherapy, and its impact on her daughter). However, even the impacts of visual disfigurement produced by the illness could be somewhat over-ridden by the presence of function. Barbara (see p. 50) *[Barbara, age 48 with cervical cancer; Dimitri, age 53—husband; Greek]*, for example, emphasised her ability to wash the dishes at the kitchen sink, rather than the extensive oedema of her lower body caused by venous and lymphatic obstruction.

Function importantly did not only incorporate physical ability, but also mental ability. The intactness of mental capacity and function was shown to be even more fundamentally important to the notion of 'self'.

The 'intuitive' emphasis

Unusual or extraordinary experiences with patients, together with the often unique way that a GP assessed an individual situation, also shaped impressions of how threatening an illness was and how the caring process was viewed. This 'intuition' or 'gut reaction' could be a powerful means of judging clinical states and expected outcomes. It could operate either independently of the epidemiological, disease burden and functional orientations to care, or it could serve to modify their emphasis. New avenues of research are finding that positive emotional well-being contributes to improved physical health (Hull, 1994). Such work is beginning to provide a tentatively acceptable (that is, scientific) foundation to positive intuitive feelings on the part of the GP, if these 'rub off' onto the patient.

'Gut reactions' could be positive or negative in relation to epidemiologically expected outcome. Positive or optimistic gut reaction tended to decline as function deteriorated and overall disease burden increased. However, positive intuitions were not exclusively confined to relatively early phases of illness—pleasant surprises were still possible in advanced illness, and, furthermore, were not necessarily rare:

THEODORE ... I think, it's a gut reaction. ... I mean, this fella had ... half his ... [paused] left lung removed. ... That was twelve years ago. Then, if you'd asked me, I would have said, ... you know, six months to nine months [to live]. Adenocarcinoma of the ... chest. ... Hundred a day smoker. [He] stopped it ... [and he's] ... fit as a bloody fiddle [today].   *[Theodore, GP, age 63; Greek]*

And again:

THEODORE ... I've been crying over one cancer patient for the last ten bloody years and she's still alive and well and came in today. ... She won't have anything done to her and she's got a massive cancer on her lungs, ... and she feels fit as a fiddle apart from the cough.   *[Theodore, GP, age 63; Greek]*

Part of such optimism was due to advances in medical management which had improved survival rates. The older practitioners could more readily relate to such advances because of their direct, first-hand comparison with older, outdated therapies. Such comparisons could be utilised to clinical advantage in reassuring very anxious patients and families:

THEODORE ... cancer's not often that deadly. The other thing is of course, say, cancer of the breast—I haven't lost a patient in fifteen years. ... It's probably coincidence ... I know we hear about how "the 'sibethera' died [of breast cancer]". ['Sibethera' is a term that parents use for their child's mother-in-law.] [I'm talking about] my own ones [i.e. breast cancer patients], I'm only talking about ten to fifteen of them, because of the improvements since the early 80s. ... So I can't think of one that has died in the last eighteen years ... because of the therapy. ... For some unknown reason they haven't relapsed. That's wonderful. So I'm very optimistic, ... compared to 1959, where they used to turn up because they'd refuse surgery and they would have cauliflower stuck on their breasts and it is the most horrendous thing. You've probably never seen one. But if you can understand a small cauliflower stuck on a breast ... and no pain.

[Theodore, GP, age 63; Greek]

Such hopeful feelings, however, did not need to be *intrinsic* to the personality or clinical experience of the doctor, but could also be *induced* by extraordinary clinical histories. The survival of Brendan *[Brendan, age mid-40s with cerebral glioma; Michelle, age ?—wife]*, for example, could not fail to produce wonder, and to therefore inject extra hope for the success of treatment in *him* (whereas such hope would *not* be present in *others* with his tumour type):

FIELD NOTES Brendan is a relatively young man in his mid-forties who had been diagnosed with primary epilepsy some sixteen years previously. Several years after this, in the 1980s, a diagnosis of a frontal lobe glioblastoma was made. A de-bulking procedure followed by radiotherapy was expected to produce only temporary palliation because of the known aggressive course of the malignancy and of the unfavourable histological appearance, which suggested maximally aggressive disease. However, he defied the odds and survived to the amazement of his doctors. His cerebral disease 'recurred' in the late 1980s with need for further therapy that again to everyone's amazement seemed to effect a cure. More recently, however, he again underwent neurosurgery for recurrent cerebral glioma ... He also had a long and complex background medical history which included the removal of a stage 3 malignant melanoma from his neck in the mid-1970s.

[Brendan, age mid-40s with cerebral glioma; Michelle, age ?—wife]

Negative intuitive feelings about illness were ubiquitous in GPs but these were not disproportionate to 'realistic' epidemiological expectation. That is, it was rare for intuition to be more negative than the anticipated epidemiological outlook. However, GP intuition was often more positive than the anticipated epidemiological outlook.

The situation in patients and families was varied. Fear of cancer could see the adoption of intensely negative outlooks. Paradoxically, however, such fear *simultaneously* drove many, especially Greek families, to the counter-acting attitude of excessive hope. An example related to the comments of Mark concerning his ill mother:

FIELD NOTES According to son Mark, the prognosis on diagnosis was "three days", then it slowly expanded to "three weeks", then "three months", and now, "who knows?"

[Paraskevi, age 48 with cervical cancer; Mark, age 23—son; Greek]

The 'chronicity' emphasis

The *chronicity* of the illness process was sometimes the main ingredient that shaped GPs' feelings and experience of palliative care, rather than the cancer's epidemiology, extent, or functional consequences. The incurability of the illness itself, and therefore its on-going chronicity, formed the main criterion of the 'palliative' nature of the care. The chronicity emphasis therefore described a mode or a mentality of *engaging* the illness—it prepared and braced the GP for an ongoing process of support.

The chronicity emphasis was independent of how fatal or non-fatal, turbulent or smooth, pleasant or unpleasant the illness itself was. Care for conditions that would not be primarily fatal in their own right, such as osteoarthritis, chronic obstructive airways disease, or persistent psychological or psychiatric disorders, thus constituted palliative care as much as did care of fatal illness:

> **ANASTASIA** ... I don't think it [i.e. palliative care] means ... the old, sort of superstitious definition that was if someone was palliative they were dying and that they were going to die. You know, I mean palliation I think can mean just adequate analgesia and adequate pain control regardless ... I mean, someone with chronic pain, you could still provide them with the sort of palliative care ... or someone with MS [i.e. multiple sclerosis] ... who's gonna be around for the next twenty years but ... they still need ... adequate ... pain control or ... other sort(s) of services, ... and that, you're only just controlling the symptoms and you're not, you're not actually changing the progression of the illness. ...
>
> *[Anastasia, GP, age 31; Greek]*

And again:

> **THEODORE** ... palliative care doesn't come in that often in cancers or terminal patients. I see it more for the arthritics, the stroke patients where there is no [cure] ... [A]rthritis of course has got severe pain ... there's a hundred arthritic patients to every one cancer. *[Theodore, GP, age 63; Greek]*

Although centred on inability to cure, this notion was not necessarily incompatible even with the attitudes of patients and carers who greatly feared cancer (Greek and Anglo-Celtic alike). That was because the chronicity approach presented families with a concerted and continuous effort at ongoing support, not a permeating attitude of 'poor prognosis' and complete resignation. The grim truth was thus associated with a sense of security:

> **MARIA** He [the GP] always spoke to us simply and ... respectfully. He would say at times, "We are trying—whatever we can." They are people who don't have hopes for me at all—within three months, I will depart. He always spoke the truth. This is ... of course maybe others don't want the truth. It didn't bother me—the truth made me happy ... I have taken it decisively.
>
> *[Maria, age 69 with breast cancer; Peter, age 74—husband; Greek]*

The 'partnership' emphasis

The concept of what palliative care was could also be centred on the interaction between doctor and patient. The *therapeutic partnership*, rather than the presence of cancer, legitimised and characterised the caring process. It could only truly exist if doctor and patient were in agreement that a long-term problem (not necessarily a fatal one) existed, and that they needed to interact closely to deal with it. Without the *mutual* consent and cooperation of both parties in a partnership, palliative care was impossible:

> **BEN** I think at some point ... in the life of the person with the illness, they find the need ... to take on a partner, a medical partner. ... And a whole series of ... negotiations then take place, often very rapidly and ... in a very fragile, precarious sort of way, but once the relationship there is made—and it's essential in agreement, to agree upon the treatment—[it's important] for the doctor to support that person, ... [and] that the person is going to work with you one way or the other ... I think the sense of ... palliative care as such is, it's as though the gate is open.
>
> *[Ben, GP, age 49; Jewish]*

And again:

> **BEN** Well, people have to allow themselves to have palliative care. And ... the aspects of denial are not necessarily removed ... ; ... certainly though ... the recognition by the patient that they are going to not only need help today but tomorrow and the next day. That their family may also need support, ... that they are going to need a guide or interpreter ... as they ... pass on towards death. I think they are the kind of [pause] events that define the beginning of the real palliative care relationship. ... And it can totally alter a pre-existing doctor–patient relationship ... from one of... maybe brevity [last word unclear] or ... relative ... dis-involvement to a completely different level. And so in effect, one way or the other, it comes about by invitation. ... It's invitation only. ... And it ... one can't force oneself into that situation and expect that it will be a stable ... arrangement ... because it inevitably is not.
>
> *[Ben, GP, age 49; Jewish]*

This was a dynamic view of palliative care because it hinged exclusively on agreement, whereas the other emphases in palliative care could operate in isolation from agreement, at least in theory. The level of *belonging* and *trust* that doctor, patient and carer felt towards each other was a key factor in the partnership emphasis. Doctors, especially those not previously well known to the patient, were often tested prior to being fully trusted:

ANASTASIA ... I'll speak to you about my ... Cyprian [fellow], ... He's seventy-three, came in with his wife who was a new patient and ... I met him in October '95 for the first time. ... And ... he said, "Oh look, we've heard you do home visits and one of our neighbours said you do home visits so I've come to see ya". I said, "Oh, okay". ... Anyway [has a drink from her cup of tea] he walked in and ... he looked a bit older than his wife and [he] ... sat down and he said, "You know, I've got diabetes and I want you to look after my diabetes". I said, "Oh, okay that's fine", you know and ... I talked about [diabetes] ... So, you know, once he sort of thought, "Okay this is the diabetes and she knows about her diabetes", he pulls out this letter from the hospital. ... Diagnosis: Burkitt's lymphoma. ...

[Anastasia, GP, age 31; Greek]

Greek patients seemed to be less strongly inclined to form intimate partnerships with their GPs, often seeing them as inferior to specialists. The comments below from Anastasia *[Anastasia, GP, age 31; Greek]* are in complete harmony with the narratives of Margarita *[Margarita, GP, age 33; Greek]*, Theodore *[Theodore, GP, age 63; Greek]*, and Andrew *[Andrew, GP, age early 40s; Greek]*:

ANASTASIA ... There are patients who really know how to use their GP as an advocate for them and they end up getting the best of care that way, ... especially I'm talking about public patients. ... I don't think Greek patients are very good at that ... , at using their GP in ... [a] sort of an advocate role and ... they tend to shop around too. ... You think if ever there ... was ever a time where they needed someone to really [get to know them well] ... now [i.e. the palliative care situation] is the time ... I think it's like ... [pause] you know, "Maybe someone else has got to offer a little bit more hope", and therefore a better outcome ... But anyway ... it becomes difficult when ... you want them to be aware that, "Hey, you're here for regular check-ups and to see how you're going", and to get to know the family and stuff.

[Anastasia, GP, age 31; Greek]

And again:

ANASTASIA ... they're not very good at seeing their GP as their advocate, or someone who can look after them in the big hospital. And I think ... it's hard to impress that on them. ... Whereas I think non-Greek-speaking patients find that a lot easier. A much easier concept to have, ... 'cause they'd rather be out of the big hospitals, ... they'd rather be looked after by their GP and rather be at home and stuff, you know. ... The younger Greek patients that I have aren't that way because they've been brought up here and have a concept of a family doctor ... whereas ... the older patients, who are the ones who are going to be sick, [don't].

[Anastasia, GP, age 31; Greek]

For a fuller harmony, partnerships also had to exist between doctor and family, as well as patient and family, as shown by Elizabeth *[Elizabeth, GP, age 32; Croatian]* when talking about an older patient with adenocarcinoma of the bowel:

ELIZABETH But it was also frustrating because you know, we [i.e. Elizabeth and her patient] had a great relationship going and, and in fact a few times the patient interrupted her daughter and said, "Look, you know, let the doctor finish what she's about to say", ... and she was actually getting annoyed by the daughter. ... The daughter would call me frequently, ... "Have you got this result in yet? Why aren't you doing this? Why aren't you doing that?"

[Elizabeth, GP, age 32; Croatian]

Further than that, partnerships were also needed between the multidisciplinary team involved in the care of the family. Dissatisfaction could arise in such partnerships on issues of communication, availability, or therapeutic effectiveness. A mutual understanding of the 'boundary' or scope of each team member was important in preventing conflict (Aldridge, 1987). Clashes in the approaches of different health–team members sometimes had destructive consequences for patient, family and health professional alike:

THEODORE ... we spent many hours talking, for example, to ... [a patient] with leukaemia, acute myeloid leukaemia, ... she was seventy-eight years of age, ... we spent a lot of time relaxing her, saying, "Look, ... you know, it could go on for years ...", and the usual, reassuring her. The next day one of the counsellors turned up and said, "You know you're going to die very quickly and you're going to get worse", and by the time they'd finished ... He'd turned up and really the next thing I knew I had this call that she was very distressed. ... You know, that's the sort of thing that distresses me when it hasn't happened once, it happened several times. ... And they have been people, not anybody, they'd been people with degrees. [Theodore, GP, age 63; Greek]

Conclusion: towards unifying patient and doctor experiences

This chapter has described the emotional landscape of the cancer world as it was lived by patients, their carers and GPs. It was within this complex landscape that medical authority or power had to be negotiated and enacted.

The cancer world of patient and carer was dominated by the task of coming to terms with the illness and the changing concept of self, as well as how to normalise life in the face of such upheaval. Although cancer illness also directly and personally threatened the GP, their cancer world was more dominated by the therapeutic emphasis and challenges that cancer posed. The therapeutic emphasis, after all, was what legitimised and defined their role and involvement with patients and families.

The respective sections dealing with each of these cancer worlds have described the *breadth* of encountered experiences. However, the experience of any given *individual* might correlate with only a small portion of such an overview or, conversely, might relate to nearly all of it. The highly variable and individual ways in which cancer was experienced and contemplated meant that the context where power was expressed and determined was universally complex and emotion-laden. Differing feelings both about the illness and its management in any given *individual* (GP, patient or carer) could be present *together*, and even *fluctuate* in their relative dominance stage by stage or even moment by moment. This paralleled the descriptions of 'oscillating movement' in the emotions of family practice residents regarding their dying patients (Dozor & Addison, 1992), and was well illustrated by the comments of Mary:

> MARY ... [it is difficult] to see your person dying ... Sometimes I see him and cut off all my hopes, sometimes I see him and I say, "Ah, he doesn't have anything, he is good now". ... This is it. ... This is the agony now ....
>
> *[Panteleimon, age 62 with lung cancer; Mary, age 63—wife; Greek]*

The particular way in which the illness situation was viewed could actually make medical power seem *paradoxical*, because power could be strongly present when disease was incurable (as when most emphasis was on function), or it could be rendered impotent in situations where the disease itself was eminently treatable (as when progress was not as good as expected). Ultimately, however, the form which medical power took, and the desirability of such a form, was a phenomenon that was shaped by *interaction* between people. In that way, medical power was *relative* because, although always socially inherent in an abstract way, it only took on 'concrete reality' in the context of lived interaction between people.

This chapter has created a basic foundation in having separately described the cancer worlds of patient/carer and GP. The next step, the building up of this foundation, is to examine the *way in which these two worlds interacted with each other*, and how such interaction shaped, determined and influenced medical power. An especially central question in such a task is how well the dynamic and complex cancer experience of a given individual could be conveyed to, and understood by, others around them. If, in aesthetic or religious experiences, emotion surpasses description with words (Good, 1994), then likewise it seems difficult to neatly circumscribe the cancer experience through the communication and negotiation that the patient-centred approach so heavily relies upon. The extent to which this is possible will therefore be a central issue in the subsequent discussion.

The next chapter will begin the task of examining the coming together of the patient/carer and clinician worlds. It presents their interaction over the entire course of the illness trajectory from initial symptoms to formal diagnosis of cancer, to subsequent phases of the illness and their management. In so doing, the *dynamics* and the *evolution* of relationships between doctor, patient and family will be studied, providing insight into how power is negotiated, enacted and expressed.

2

Doctor–family interaction

The preceding chapter has shown that adjusting to, and coping with, the presence of cancer was a dominant issue in the world of patients and carers. Doctors could view the illness more objectively or dispassionately, and so the medical world revolved around the management possibilities that the illness presented.

Both of these worlds, however, *encountered* each other and *interacted* with each other. It is this encounter over the course of the illness that forms the focus of the present chapter. Important stages in the illness trajectory were defined by key terms such as 'diagnosis', 'treatment', 'remission', 'cure', 'relapse' and 'dying', showing that it was essentially a 'status passage' (Glaser & Strauss, 1971). This passage began at 'normality' and proceeded in variable directions. Box 2.1 on page 64 shows such sequences in the informants.

Key events in cancer illness were characterised by major *change,* either in illness site and extent, interpersonal relationships, social status, family circumstances, or personal attitudes. These were the most sensitive and delicate periods of the illness trajectory. Even though the illness was experienced as a *continuous whole,* it was these critical periods of change that were greatly amplified in people's feelings and memories. They challenged medical power according to how severe, predictable and controllable they were.

Despite the individuality of the illness experience, the patient, carer and GP narratives generally concurred in their definitions of critical periods and key tasks in the illness. However, that did not ensure uniformity in the *type* of emphasis given *within* a given critical issue. For

BOX 2.1 Sequences of illness progression

PATTERN 1	Seen in:
ill at diagnosis	• [Maria, age 69 with breast cancer; Peter, age 74—husband; Greek],
↓	• [Aristotle, age 79 with prostate cancer;
controlled illness (steady state*)	Paula, age ?—daughter; Greek],
↓	• [Charles, age 72 with prostate cancer;
deterioration	Amanda, age 72—wife; Anglo-Celtic],
	• [Monica, age 48 with breast cancer; Alan, age late 50s—husband; Anglo-Celtic]
	• [Barbara, age 48 with cervical cancer; Dimitri, age 53—husband; Greek]

PATTERN 2	Seen in:
ill at diagnosis	• [Paraskevi, age 48 with cervical cancer; Mark, age 23—son; Greek]
↓	
controlled illness (steady state*)	

PATTERN 3	Seen in:
ill at diagnosis	• [George, age mid-50s with lung cancer; Katerina, age ?—wife; Greek],
↓	• [Clare, age 65 with stomach cancer;
deterioration	Michael, age 67—husband; Anglo-Celtic],
	• [Panteleimon, age 62 with lung cancer; Mary, age 63—wife; Greek]

PATTERN 4	Seen in:
well at diagnosis	• [Jane, English, age 61 with mycosis fungoides; John, German, age 70— husband],
↓	• [Simon, age 64 with lymphoma; Cynthia,
controlled illness (steady state*)	age 52—wife; Anglo-Celtic]
↕	
deterioration	

PATTERN 5	Seen in:
well at diagnosis	• [Brendan, age mid-40s with cerebral glioma; Michelle, age ?—wife]
↓	
controlled illness (steady state*)	
↓	
apparent cure	
↓	
deterioration	
↓	
controlled illness	

(* note that in the 'steady state', the patient's condition could be either good, average or poor) example, disclosure was a universally accepted key task, but views on its optimal timing and execution differed. The following sections examine critical illness periods and tasks. Although discussed separately, each phase affected how subsequent phases were experienced, and how preceding phases were remembered.

The pre-consultation period

This period denotes the time before a medical visit was initiated. Here, the patient and/or family assessed the symptoms for their severity, possible significance, and their response to home-based remedies. Although such periods could also occur *after* the cancer diagnosis was made, attention here is on the pre-diagnosis period.

Everyone functions below the ideal state of perfect health, yet not everyone is defined as ill (Twaddle, 1974). British surveys show that only five per cent of the general community did *not* experience illness symptoms over a two week period (Wandsworth, Butterfield & Blaney, 1971, cited in Fraser, 1992). Normal health is thus defined from a range of states that indicate 'less than perfect' health (Twaddle, 1974). Consistent with this, every patient informant had *symptom thresholds* beyond which external help was needed to manage them.

The process leading to medical presentation did *not* necessarily involve a detailed and elaborate weighing-up of the threat of illness versus the need to present to the doctor, unlike the theorising of the Health Belief Model and related models as discussed in the Introduction:

CHARLES ... I had noticed that I wasn't passing water as easily as I used to, but like most ah stupid old people, you know, I sort of thought, "Oh, it'll come good", you know. But unfortunately, it didn't.
[Charles, age 72 with prostate cancer; Amanda, age 72—wife; Anglo-Celtic]

Sometimes, significant symptoms came to the doctor's attention incidentally, and not in a planned manner. Elizabeth *[Elizabeth, GP, age 32; Croatian]*, for example, recalled one patient who told her about blood in her stools just as they were leaving the room after completing a routine consultation. On inspection, an anal carcinoma was discovered. Hope that symptoms were not dangerous could exist in tension with symptoms which were *known* to be potentially life-threatening. That indicated an internal, personal struggle for control and normality:

INTERVIEWER ... At the beginning, you said that there was a, a period where you had warning bells ... but you let it pass for a while ... Why had you decided not to pursue it, Monica?

MONICA I think ... two things. ... I'm probably like everyone else and wanted to believe that everything was fine. ... I think the other thing ... I'd been working on training science, and in fact one of the jobs that I did was to go through all the breast cancer files from the research reports. ... And I think I had firmly convinced myself at that stage that if your breast feeding was of a very natural, on-demand sort of breast feeding ... that statistically ... you didn't get breast cancer. ... Now, I know that ... for every statistical truth, there are the aberrations, ... the ones who lie outside. ... And I guess, I chose not to remember that. ... So I guess that that fed a bit my wish to feel, you know, everything's all right ...

[Monica, age 48 with breast cancer; Alan, age late 50s—husband; Anglo-Celtic]

Hope could also temper a situation that *definitely was* adverse. Monica *[Monica, age 48 with breast cancer; Alan, age late 50s—husband; Anglo-Celtic]*, for example, maintained hope when her illness relapsed after chemotherapy and surgery. This hope, however, was altered or revised. Prior to diagnosis it was hope that the illness was not serious. After diagnosis, it was hope for a cure. After cure seemed remote, it was hope for a good quality of life.

Symptoms deemed significant often led the patient to a stepwise recruitment of people to assist if self-initiated actions failed. Disclosures therefore occurred in *grades*. Family members were often made aware directly (that is, verbally), but sometimes indirectly through the patient's altered function or interaction. Ultimately, the persistence of a problem led to a medical consultation.

The medical diagnostic process

Diagnosis of cancer or its complications occurred in different ways. It could be based on symptoms and signs, or tests, or both. It could also occur in the process of *treatment*, as with Aristotle *[Aristotle, age 79 with prostate cancer; Paula, age ?—daughter; Greek]*, where trans-urethrally resected prostate tissue unexpectedly proved to be malignant. The degree to which the diagnosis was expected was thus variable.

Successful diagnosis engendered confidence in the doctor and was therefore a pivotal test of medical power. However, diagnosis had many inherent challenges and uncertainties, especially in general practice, where illness often presented early and therefore in a poorly differentiated state.

Gross morbid pathology as illustrated in classic surgical textbooks was thus only rarely encountered. Instead, symptoms and signs were often difficult to *label* and biomedically *define*. 'Vague' symptomatology (perceived by Greek GPs to be prominent among their Greek patients) generated a long list of differential diagnoses that caused difficulty for the GPs.

Although poor communication by the doctor is a key cause of patient dissatisfaction, too much honest expression of uncertainty in defining the symptomatology could cause unnecessary concern, engender mistrust in the doctor, and affect continuity of care and compliance with treatment. The GP's best course of action was often based on common-sense clinical acumen, and probabilities had to be balanced. Sometimes *time* and *observation* were used as diagnostic tools. Medical investigations could be useful but the potential for false-positive or false-negative results could wreak emotional havoc on both patient and doctor alike (Vafiadis, 1996).

Despite this, patient and carer expectations in diagnostic medicine were often high, reinforced by the powerful images of complicated instruments or gadgetry that were used in testing procedures. The failure of doctors to diagnose early therefore caused a *lasting* perplexity in some families. Maria's metastatic breast cancer, for example, was not detected by initial tests; not believing it could have been missed, Maria felt that her Greek GP had withheld the truth:

> **MARIA** … You couldn't draw any conclusions about it [i.e. about the GP not telling her it was cancer] at the time. Didn't he know [what the matter was]? Didn't he wish [to disclose it]? Did he feel sorry [for me]? … I put it down to him feeling sorry for me, … because I had all the tests … Let him not say, "You have cancer", let him say to me, "Your blood is sick, and we can help it", or, "I will change your medications to different ones". …
>
> **PETER** He was saying to us that all was well. …
>
> **INTERVIEWER** The other thing is that the illness might not have progressed to the point of showing up on the tests, and the tests were OK then, who knows?
>
> **MARIA** But they weren't … He didn't find it in the breast—he didn't pay attention to this. But the blood? But the examinations? … The X-rays … of the leg? … He should have helped in some way …
>
> *[Maria, age 69 with breast cancer; Peter, age 74—husband; Greek]*

Such disappointment may have been eased if the significance of Maria's symptoms had been acknowledged. Instead, normal test results somewhat dismissed them. It generally seemed that such *pre-disclosures* (that is, official medical recognition of a significant but as yet undefined problem), together with efforts to clarify the problem, were universally important to patients and families.

Naming the condition especially helped the definition and psychological encapsulation of the problem (Good, 1994). That was particularly striking with Jane, who had years of empirical therapy before her cancer type became recognised within the general body of medical knowledge:

> **JANE** But he still hadn't given me a name to it. ... Yes but it wasn't until I was about twenty-six [pause] the ... Victorian Hospital sent me to Dr Simpson, Simpson sent me to James. James G. ... at St Vincent's. ... And I said, "What is this?" What is the *name* [emphasised] for this condition? And he said, "You have a condition by the name of mycosis fungoides". Well, at least I'd got a name.
> *[Jane, English, age 61 with mycosis fungoides; John, German, age 70—husband]*

Naming the condition, however, did not always bring such relief. The incidental or unexpected diagnosis was usually devastating, plunging the patient and family into the world of cancer and imprinting itself into their lives and memories:

> **FIELD NOTES** He stood in the hallway as he told her [of his cancer diagnosis], and Cynthia stated very vividly that to this day, whenever she looks down the hallway, she recalls that day seven years ago when Simon told her.
> *[Simon, age 64 with lymphoma; Cynthia, age 52—wife; Anglo-Celtic]*

Unexpected diagnoses occurred in several ways. The history and examination sometimes suggested the diagnosis to the doctor but it remained unexpected to the patient and family. The diagnosis could follow a routine screening procedure such as a Papanicolaou smear, mammography, a skin check, or some such other (none of the patients here belonged to this category, which awaits further research). The diagnosis could also follow assessment for what seemed a non-threatening illness to both patient and doctor alike, and could be either related or unrelated to the presenting symptoms. Simon's case *[Simon, age 64 with lymphoma; Cynthia, age 52—wife; Anglo-Celtic]* was an example, where neither he nor his doctors expected that the excised lymph node from his neck would reveal non-Hodgkin's lymphoma.

The unexpected diagnosis itself did not usually challenge the credibility of medicine, since medicine had done its job by defining the problem. Medicine, however, faced major challenges in dealing with subsequent phases of the illness. Some of these challenges are now considered in more detail.

The nature and purpose of disclosure

In disclosure, the palliative care literature often focuses on the initial revelation of the cancer diagnosis by the doctor to the patient and family. This time heralds an enormous transition into the realm of serious illness. Important disclosures, however, also occurred *throughout* the illness. Illness relapse, the need for chemotherapy, a blood transfusion, or morphine could all be as emotionally significant as the initial revelation of cancer itself, effectively equating to a *second* cancer diagnosis. That was especially so if previous progress had been positive. Disclosures could also be positive and could ease emotional anguish, even if they were not major. For example, a slowing of illness progression could be very welcome news. *Relative* gains were thus often more important than absolute ones.

Disclosure had practical purposes (such as improving patients' involvement and compliance with treatment), moral purposes (concerning people's right to 'know') and emotional purposes (in sharing burdens with others). However, despite these supposed advantages, the level of awareness that patients and their carers had of the cancer illness was often less than complete.

Awareness in disclosure

The American norm in the 1960s to conceal bad news from the terminal patient (Glaser & Strauss, 1965) reflected society's pre-occupation with the *biology* of death, not its complete denial (Kellehear, 1984). Subsequent emphasis on patient-centredness saw a more open, early disclosure of terminal illness established as the norm. Despite this, however, recent estimates suggest that between only forty-four to sixty-six per cent of dying patients know that their illness is fatal (Kellehear, 1990). A spectrum of awareness was also seen in patients and families in this study, ranging from scant to highly detailed.

The ideal of 'full disclosure' did not always happen because of the emotive nature of cancer and the complex nature of awareness. Glaser and Strauss (1965) pointed to such complexity through their descriptions of different awareness contexts in terminally ill hospital patients (Box 2.2 on page 70).

BOX 2.2 Awareness contexts in terminal illness (after Glaser & Strauss, 1965)

Closed awareness	Patient unaware of diagnosis or prognosis.
Suspected awareness	Patient suspects the diagnosis or prognosis but does not seek or receive confirmation.
Mutual-pretence awareness	All parties recognise the situation but 'pretend' it is not there.
Open awareness	All parties know the diagnosis and acknowledge it openly.
Discounted awareness	The awareness of one party is discounted totally by others (e.g. with demented patients).

Although all informants to this study believed in the necessity of disclosure, views on its optimal timing, method and content differed. Further, awareness or non-awareness could relate to many *different aspects* of the *same* illness, pointing to the limitations in the model depicted in Box 2.2. For example, the patient who is aware of their diagnosis but *not* their fatal prognosis would simultaneously belong to the open and closed awareness contexts, and also quite possibly to the suspected awareness and mutual-pretence awareness contexts as well.

Kellehear (1990) addressed this complexity through studying awareness of cancer and dying exclusively from the patient's perspective. He noted the importance of suspicion as a *preliminary form* of awareness, and highlighted the importance that the stage of illness had in setting the context within which awareness was enacted. Awareness of diagnosis therefore differed from awareness of prognosis, and their relative timing became important, since they might occur together or be separated by varying periods of time (Kellehear, 1990). Awareness of a terminal diagnosis, where death was located at some future point, also differed in quality from the awareness of being near that actual point itself (Kellehear, 1990).

In the developed world, 'the overwhelming source of awareness remains the doctor' (Kellehear, 1990: 84). Despite the doctrine of informed consent, Miyaji (1993) in the United States observed that hospital doctors differed in their views of what patients 'want to know' versus 'what they need to know'. This offered doctors potential flexibility in the completeness of disclosure. This was also the case of GPs in this study. Even GPs most oriented to disclosing the 'full' truth displayed flexibility in their approaches, such as a willingness not to disclose unless openly asked, or unless it became absolutely necessary. The content and method of GPs' disclosures depended on how they felt the patient and family would cope, how they themselves were coping, and also on practical issues such as time availability and the conduciveness of the setting. Some GPs welcomed the patient's right to forgo full disclosure, while others sometimes left disclosure to others:

BYRON ... 'if they don't ask, you don't tell' is sometimes a good rule but, ... you can answer pretty matter-of-factly in vague terms. ... You want to spare them any extra anxieties and fears. ... And ... indeed, the less tense they are, the less pain they're feeling. *[Byron, GP, age 57; Anglo-Celtic]*

And again:

INTERVIEWER ... Let's move on to disclosing the problem.
THEODORE That is a difficult problem. ... And I'm a coward [laughs], so I'll let ... other people disclose it; my specialist—what, what are they being paid for? They get more money than I do. [laughs] ... I don't like giving bad news.
[Theodore, GP, age 63; Greek]

GP disclosures often emphasised the *currently good aspects* of the illness rather than its inevitable *future bad aspects*. Attaining the right balance in emphasis was, however, often complicated. Andrew, for example, reflected on the encouragement that specialists gave to many cancer patients currently in remission but who had a high risk of relapsing:

ANDREW ... you feel really good for them but you know deep down ... in a few months it's not really going to be great and you will be back here and you're going to say to me, "How come?" ... So how do we address that? What do we say to them? I mean, do we shatter their hopes? ... You have to be supporting the patient and giving them hope because if they're positive you know that they've got better outcomes. ... So you've got to fight against being negative but then you've also got to be realistic . ... That's difficult. *[Andrew, GP, age early 40s; Greek]*

Even negative news, however, could be optimised. Bad news could still contain some positive direction (such as a plan of action, however modest, to alleviate symptoms). The unpredictability of the illness could be advantageously used to emphasise the uncertainty of future *negative* progress, rather than the uncertainty of future positive progress. A demonstrated commitment to the patient could also dull the effect of bad news. All of these factors showed that disclosure could be converted into a therapeutic tool, even when the news was bad:

MARIA ... if we say that we will live [forever], it is impossible. ... That's how man is made—he will go [i.e. die] from something. ... And the doctor is human. He goes in with an effort, he goes with a certain hope, to save from bad outcomes, but ... only that there must exist an, an honesty, [and] to convey a sense of courage, so that the doctor naturally does not leave a sense of gloom upon a person.

[Maria, age 69 with breast cancer; Peter, age 74—husband; Greek]

Dynamics of disclosure

Four key points were noted about the dynamics of disclosure, relating to its source, direction and sequence, timing and multiplicity.

Source of disclosure

Doctors were not the only *source* of disclosure in cancer illness, a point not emphasised enough in the palliative care literature. Relatives, friends or other health professionals were important sources of awareness for patients (Kellehear, 1990). Patients and their carers were also important disclosure sources, especially regarding illness progress and response to treatment (through descriptions of their symptoms).

Direction and sequence in disclosure

Disclosure had *direction* and *sequence* (see Figure 2.1). Information could pass through various people in different orders before reaching the final destination. Different persons, often within families, could therefore receive news at different times. The final destination of the news may or may not have been intended.

FIGURE 2.1 Possible directions in disclosure

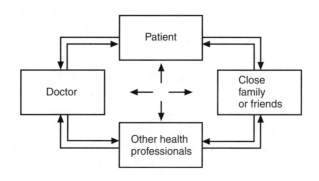

Disclosure sometimes came from *two or more sources* (simultaneously or separately), or was delivered to two or more types of recipient. Information was sometimes *filtered* by the person disclosing it, often consciously, sometimes unconsciously. Because of that, information at the end of the relay system could vary considerably from what was disclosed originally.

Greek families tended to shield the patient from bad news, whereas a more open context reigned in Anglo-Celtic families. The frequent inability of the Greek patient to speak English facilitated filtering, which often involved selective withholding of information, rather than its falsification:

> **PAULA** ... Probably he didn't realise it [i.e. the cancer diagnosis] so much, we didn't tell him. ... He knew it but, let's say, he didn't ... I think that he didn't understand it so much.
>
> *[Aristotle, age 79 with prostate cancer; Paula, age ?—daughter; Greek]*

GPs faced a dilemma when asked by families to participate in filtering or falsifying of information. While their training acknowledged the primacy of the patient, GPs often complied with the family's wishes *if* they fell within the GP's own *ethical boundaries*. The decision of the family to withhold information from the patient was sometimes deemed appropriate. However, many GPs drew the line at lying to the patient or concealing information when it was specifically requested. Some Greek patients themselves distanced the illness by not seeking in-depth information about it, or repelling it when it was forthcoming, as seen with George *[George, age mid-50s with lung cancer; Katerina, age ?—wife; Greek].* That allowed them to maintain some *control* over the situation.

On the whole, it was uncommon for a Greek patient to actively protect and comfort their family. Anglo-Celtic patients, however, often withheld illness details from the family: they were more often the protector rather than the protected:

> **MONICA** Alan still does [experience difficulties in coping]. I mean, this morning he was a bit of a mess, because I'd just gone the day before yesterday to the oncologist, ... rung Alan at work, [and] said, "Oh, I've got a bit of fluid on the lung, I've got to have it drained. Oh well, can you drive me in on ... Thursday?", and then told him to pick me up. And that's how I have to deal with it. ... I have to be a bit mechanical. ... He was a bit stroppy this morning and ... I just said,

"Hey, you've got to stop worrying when I have these things. Think of it as me taking a Panadol".

[Monica, age 48 with breast cancer; Alan, age late 50s—husband; Anglo-Celtic]

Timing of disclosure

Disclosure in a *graded fashion over time* was often favoured over full, open and immediate disclosure:

PAULA Yeah, we told him because ... he had to have ... radiotherapy. ... In the beginning it was true that we didn't want to tell him but as you can understand it is preferable for him to know because he is having therapy, and often if you hear about and know that you are having that sort of therapy, you have this sort of illness [i.e. cancer].

[Aristotle, age 79 with prostate cancer; Paula, age ?—daughter; Greek]

However, grading of disclosure ran the risk of delaying it too long. In such cases, the patient's increasing suspicion of secrecy led to distrust in the family and doctor. This was seen with Paraskevi [*Paraskevi, age 48 with cervical cancer; Mark, age 23—son; Greek*].

Disclosure thus occurred in a setting of *knowledge* and *counter-knowledge*. The person disclosing the news, or the recipient, or both, usually had some background knowledge or impressions about the condition or what the other party knew about it. Such counter-knowledge was used as a mirror against which incoming knowledge was reflected and tested for compatibility. A patient with severe, intractable symptoms would therefore be suspicious of statements that they would get well soon.

Multiplicity in disclosure

Disclosures could be made *multiple times* by the same person (for example, the GP in reinforcing the facts, or raising them again in response to questions), or a given person could receive the same disclosure from different parties (such as different members of the multidisciplinary team). The emotional fragility of the process at the one-to-one level was greatly magnified when many persons were involved, because each viewed the problem from their own perspective. This created the potential for conflicting information, and thus confusion and distress. A striking example of this was given by Theodore [*Theodore, GP, age 63; Greek*], in which the potentially negative implications of the multidisciplinary model were made clear (see p. 60).

Emotive and non-verbal content of disclosure

Health professionals, patients and families often shared intensely personal issues not directly concerning the cancer pathology itself. For the GP, however, a suitable person before whom they could 'open up' was not always at hand. Sharing feelings with the patient and their family was not always appropriate, especially if the GP was not coping emotionally. Carol's *[Carol, GP, age mid-30s; Anglo-Celtic]* narrative showed that even the GP's own spouse might be unsuitable to share certain feelings with because they might not understand the context which generated the difficulty.

Non-verbal components associated with either receiving or providing a disclosure (or, conversely, of *not* receiving or providing it) both expressed and added to its emotion. Mannerisms, periods of silence, rising medication dosages, progression of symptoms, or increasing frequency of medical attention could be as powerful as verbal disclosures and often braced the person for verbal confirmation of the worst. This was seen with Michael's wait for the results of a staging laparotomy on his wife:

> **MICHAEL** Well then we ... walked up to the operating theatre ... as far as we could go, and we came back and we went down and had a coffee ... They said it was going to be about two hours or more and she was only away about an hour and a quarter and ... she come back. And I thought, "God, this is bad", you know. And then the sister came out and said, "Oh, ... Professor wants to talk to you", ... but ... he didn't come down; ... the register general [i.e. registrar] was there ... and she came and spoke to us ... and told us ... that ... it was no good, ... they didn't do anything, ... they said as soon as they opened it [i.e. the abdomen], it [i.e. the cancer] was too far back.
>
> *[Clare, age 65 with stomach cancer; Michael, age 67—husband; Anglo-Celtic]*

Should disclosure focus primarily on knowledge or on coping?

Key disclosures such as diagnosis, relapse or remission had *permanent* repercussions on all future emotions and outlooks in the illness. Varying individual preferences, and the complex dynamics of disclosure and awareness made it difficult to prescribe an ideal disclosure method for clinical use. The legalistic, textbook consensus of always conveying 'the truth' seemed simplistic and could be destructive. One hospice, seeing how much Panteleimon *[Panteleimon, age 62 with lung cancer; Mary, age*

63—wife; Greek] was incapacitated by his diagnosis, concluded that open disclosure had been inappropriate—a conclusion at odds with current palliative care philosophy. This showed that neglecting the 'how', 'if', 'when' and 'in what context' reduced disclosure to a concrete rule of 'telling' that was as rational, cold and impersonal as any scientific procedure ever could be.

Here, as in other studies (Gordon, 1990; Miyaji, 1993), medical disclosure of bad news usually tried to harmonise discourse about the illness with people's lived experience of it (Saillant, 1990). It was not *absolute* knowledge of the illness that disclosure sought, but rather a knowledge that would facilitate *coping* with the illness, by the doctor as well as the patient. The 'bio-psycho-social' model of total care (Engel, 1977) had to be used to *construct* a vision of optimal care, rather than becoming *superimposed* on pre-existing visions of such care. Such a construction necessitated re-framing the basic issue of disclosure away from the common 'knowing' versus 'not knowing' dichotomy. Alternative paradigms included the active induction or use of intermediate levels of knowledge, or the careful balancing of positive and negative content in disclosure. Clinical uncertainty could also be used to emphasise uncertainty about bad outcomes, rather than uncertainty about good outcomes. The growing body of medical research showing the connection between positive emotions and enhanced physical prognosis (see. Hull, 1994) also lends objective validity to such paradigms. The difficulty in the multidisciplinary setting, however, lay in synchronising individual approaches.

Treatment as 'active' or 'passive'

Chapter 1 discussed different GP perspectives of the palliative care process. How did these marry with patient and carer views on the process of treatment?

Patients and carers understood treatment according to how 'active' or 'passive' it was, not on whether it was 'curative' or 'palliative'. Although the 'active-passive' framework incorporated the important notions of 'curable' versus 'not curable', it extended and personalised them. Although active care could be defined as care that could cure, it also referred to care that effectively alleviated symptoms. It could even apply to care that could not effectively help symptoms but which reflected a genuine effort and concern in those who administered it. Conversely, potentially curative care or care that could achieve good palliation might be seen as 'non-active' (or 'passive') if it was applied unenthusiastically, or without due consideration to other, perhaps more effective, treatment options.

Four features seemed to best define the 'active-passive' system of understanding. These related to the doctor's enthusiasm and concern, the treatment's complexity and invasiveness, the rapidity of instigating treatment, and the degree of medical certainty accompanying the treatment decision. These are now considered in more detail.

Medical enthusiasm and concern

Medical enthusiasm and concern imparted a sense of trust and confidence that positively transformed the way families viewed their illness, *irrespective* of whether or not medicine could cure it. It also made doctor–patient relationships more warm and intimate. For example, although highly satisfied with her hospital surgeons, Maria had a particular affinity with the GP who originally diagnosed her cancer, and expanded on why that was so:

> **MARIA** Well, I thought that his general air, his movements, that it was like he wanted to offer you something more [than usual care]. … It was like he was giving you a lot of interest, like he wanted to help you … very easily [last two words translated precisely; the meaning is that the doctor was offering help very freely and liberally].
>
> *[Maria, age 69 with breast cancer; Peter, age 74—husband; Greek]*

The doctor's enthusiasm could also sustain patient trust and confidence even if the doctor–patient relationship wasn't particularly warm or intimate, as seen with Jane:

> **JANE** Well, I don't think it [i.e. her liking of the doctor] was really personal, I don't think it was because he liked me … it was his curiosity, his, his desire for knowledge of the complaint. … And … the different aspects of it, and how it … especially in me … seeing it was … a variant, I obviously was reacting differently to everybody else. … That unsettled him; he wanted, he wanted answers …
>
> *[Jane, English, age 61 with mycosis fungoides; John, German, age 70—husband]*

Because it could *convert* seemingly 'passive' treatment into 'active' treatment, medical enthusiasm was a phenomenon that had considerable clinical potential.

Complexity and invasiveness of treatment

Often, the *complexity* and *invasiveness* of treatment were important markers of how 'active' it was seen to be, especially if such treatment led to improvement. However, improvement was not the decisive factor—the observation could still apply even if treatment was unhelpful. Why? Because major or dramatic interventions were more heavily *imprinted into the consciousness* of individuals and occupied a more central place in their illness narratives. In that regard, hospitals and specialists, who administered 'big' or 'important' treatments like chemotherapy, radiotherapy, or surgery, were seen as prominent sources of active care. They *tried* things; they were actually doing, or capable of doing, *major* things to people. In comparison, the GP was often seen as subservient to the specialist:

> **ANASTASIA** ... you often hear ... our 'relos' or the friends who say, "Oh, I saw the professor, he is the best!" [spoken in Greek; both laugh] ... and you think, "Oh, right, okay ... I've never heard of this Prof but hey, he must be good!", you know [sarcastically] or [they say], "I saw the Collins Street specialist", ... you know what I mean? *[Anastasia, GP, age 31; Greek]*

Hopes in advanced or complex treatment led patients to significant sacrifices, including loss of hair and nausea through chemotherapy, and complications of major surgery. The notion of 'preserving the whole person' was so powerful that patients sometimes risked losing it entirely with aggressive and life-threatening treatment.

More practical but less advanced interventions could also be seen as active, especially after the failure of more complex modalities. In comparison, however, their scope was more limited and thus they usually generated less excitement and enthusiasm. Maria *[Maria, age 69 with breast cancer; Peter, age 74—husband; Greek]*, for example, could not fully appreciate the active home surveillance and preventive work of regular nursing visits, because she was physically independent in basic self-care tasks.

Rapidity of treatment

The *rapidity* of instigating treatment also affected how 'active' the therapy was seen to be. Rapid attention optimised chances for cure and showed that the medical profession cared for the patient:

> **MARIA** ... I still think to this day ... that he [i.e. the diagnosing GP] is ... my saviour. ... He was the first doctor [to diagnose it]. He didn't put me to much

trouble, I wasn't wearied with, "Come tomorrow, come the following day", ...
[I had] therapy—within three days ... I was operated on.

[Maria, age 69 with breast cancer; Peter, age 74—husband; Greek]

The desire for rapid action, however, sometimes meant that patients had to forgo any input into such treatment decisions if the situation was urgent:

CHARLES And ... he just explained to me that if I didn't have it operated on I'd ... pass out [i.e. die] very quickly, so I decided to have the operation.

[Charles, age 72 with prostate cancer; Amanda, age 72—wife; Anglo-Celtic]

Concern about cancer from patient and family generally meant that such rapid action was ideal and welcomed, as encapsulated by Monica's statement '... *I guess at that stage I just wanted something to happen quickly'* *[Monica, age 48 with breast cancer; Alan, age late 50s—husband; Anglo-Celtic].* But that desire was closely linked to the level of medical certainty in the value of the proposed treatment.

Medical certainty and decisiveness as markers of therapeutic potential

The advantages that medical concern and rapidity lent to treatment became stifled if the proposed treatment did not stand out as the most valuable option. Monica's oncologist, for example, told her that mastectomy was not proven in reducing the mortality or morbidity of her particular condition, yet her surgeon was keen to proceed after her chemotherapy without discussing the pros and cons:

MONICA ... And oh, he read the riot act! He didn't want me to have 'radio' because you didn't heal afterwards and ... the lump was so big that ah he'd have to do a radical [resection] and he'd take flaps of skin from round the back of my ribcage and swing them round here and he was ... in the full swing of how wonderful he was and what he'd do! [expressed with powerful emotion; after a few seconds Monica regains her calm composure]. I left, went back to see my oncologist ... and said ah, "I never want to ... go near that man again".

[Monica, age 48 with breast cancer; Alan, age late 50s—husband; Anglo-Celtic]

Grey areas in medical knowledge about ideal management were not always as well understood or appreciated by patients and families, especially the Greek informants. In that sense, offering the patient or family a say in management sometimes caused *perplexity* either because it showed the medical profession to be less decisive and certain than expected, or because the patient or family felt unqualified to undertake management decisions. Maria *[Maria, age 69 with breast cancer; Peter, age 74—husband; Greek]* was an example of the latter. Although appreciative, she refused to be involved in decision-making, delegating it back to her trusted doctors. Such trust was often blind and *inherent*, especially among the older Anglo-Celtic informants, who did not question the doctor even if they did not understand what was said (as with Clare *[Clare, age 65 with stomach cancer; Michael, age 67—husband; Anglo-Celtic]*). Often, however, such trust had to be *earned*:

> **CAROL** ... he became quite psychotic and ... did all sorts of bizarre things, but one of the things he did was he climbed naked into a tree in the back garden ... I think that was the turning point of our relationship with him and his family, because ... the family were completely unable to cope and ... the patient was out of control ... and the nurse came in and settled the situation down ... and from that day forward ... they accepted our intervention and had much more confidence ...
>
> *[Carol, GP, age mid-30s; Anglo-Celtic]*

The 'activity' of non-medical forms of treatment

Simple conversations, walking, helping with basic tasks of daily living, the offering of food or drink, home remedies, the use of vitamins, and spiritual care were all important, *active* expressions of treatment or caring. GPs often tried to incorporate them as adjuvants to the medical therapy, although such attempts had to be *appropriate* to the situation. Maria's *[Maria, age 69 with breast cancer; Peter, age 74—husband; Greek]* original Greek GP, for example, encouraged her to seek a warmer climate for her 'rheumatism', but she felt too ill for that to be a realistic option.

Food intake was a very important form of supportive treatment and a criterion by which the illness was monitored. It was one of the often few things that the family could readily offer the patient. Even small offerings in advanced illness therefore took on enormous importance and became an 'active' means of assistance:

PANTELEIMON [pauses]. ... [I ate little] more than one olive, ... The days passed like that, a sip of milk, an olive. ... "Food, food", [says] the wife. ... The wife is keeping me alive. ... *[Panteleimon, age 62 with lung cancer; Mary, age 63—wife; Greek]*

Because Panteleimon *[Panteleimon, age 62 with lung cancer; Mary, age 63—wife; Greek]* could not eat much in his advanced illness, the untouched biscuits and other foodstuffs next to his bed became a powerfully dramatic and tragic symbol of a struggle that was being lost. That, however, only increased the need of the family to offer *something*, to help in some way. The untouched food, although distressing, affirmed the family's ongoing role as carers. In this light, medical control of nausea and vomiting took on a huge importance.

Other techniques also enhanced the sense of 'activity' in treatment. The use of cupping was seen in one Greek household, while acupuncture and Chinese medicine were used by several Anglo-Celtic families. Monica *[Monica, age 48 with breast cancer; Alan, age late 50s—husband; Anglo-Celtic]* felt that acupuncture and massage got *'[her] body into a healthier state so that [her] immune system can be strong'*, thereby augmenting conventional therapy, although she also felt a need for properly conducted trials to demonstrate their effectiveness.

Synchronising the notions of 'activity' and 'passivity' in treatment

The notion of 'activity' and 'passivity' in treatment was a potential tool that could facilitate the understanding of another's experience of cancer, and so optimise the treatment. However, the complex dynamics of treatment hampered the process of synchronising between the various players exactly what was 'active' and what was 'passive' in management. The more people that were involved, the more difficult things became, especially in the case of Greeks with a *very* extended family:

THEODORE ... You're quite likely to get a call from Greece saying, "My second cousin who I grew up with, what the hell's the trouble?" ...

[Theodore, GP, age 63; Greek]

Lack of agreement as to the best management approach sometimes drove patients or their families to the phenomenon of role-forcing (Glaser

& Strauss, 1965), where the doctor was directed to perform their medical role more efficiently according to the patient or family's conception of it:

> **ELIZABETH** ... The daughter would call me frequently, ... "Have you got this result in yet? Why aren't you doing this? Why aren't you doing that?"
>
> *[Elizabeth, GP, age 32; Croatian]*

More generally, however, a synchronisation of views was *facilitated* when patients and families involved themselves in medical treatment and gained knowledge of it. That imparted a sense of *control* and enhanced cooperation. Monica *[Monica, age 48 with breast cancer; Alan, age late 50s—husband; Anglo-Celtic]*, for example, being highly educated, could name her chemotherapy drugs, knew the histopathological details of her tissue biopsies, and was centrally involved in treatment decision-making. Simon and Cynthia *[Simon, age 64 with lymphoma; Cynthia, age 52—wife; Anglo-Celtic]* also distinguished their medications and chemotherapy drugs (although by colour rather than by name) according to their specific purpose.

The degree to which the GP was able or willing to accommodate patient and family views was important. This varied according to the personality of the GP, but could also change over time according to the particulars of each individual case. Sometimes GP flexibility was minimal, so that patients' non-compliance was unconsciously viewed by the GP as a fault (recall the comments of Margarita *[Margarita, GP, age 33; Greek]* in Chapter 1). At other times, flexibility allowed GPs some psychological room to work constructively around non-ideal treatment circumstances:

> **THEODORE** ... I've always gone into lifestyle, change of lifestyle, and have I been ... successful? Nobody changes lifestyle [laughs]. After the second heart attack they might stop smoking if you're lucky.   *[Theodore, GP, age 63; Greek]*

Monitoring of progress

Monitoring of illness, both *what* was monitored and *how* it was monitored, varied between people and also changed for individuals over time. Seven key modalities of monitoring, not mutually exclusive to each other, were observed as follows.

Functional monitoring

Functional status was an important monitoring modality because it was externally manifest. Good function was not only practical but, psychologically, also equated to well-being. However, what defined good functioning was *relative* to the stage of progress. In advanced illness there was great satisfaction in controlling progressively more basic aspects of existence that might otherwise be taken for granted, such as the ability to eat or to remain pain-free. Clare, for example, was greatly satisfied at being able to walk a few metres:

MICHAEL ... But she's getting so darn weak now, that's the trouble ... you see, ... and she's ... noticing that ... She stood up there [at the kitchen table] and ... I said, "Where are you going, love?" and she said, "I just want to see how far I can go", ... you know. And ... Clare walked out to there, you know [i.e. to the kitchen door, a distance of only three metres or so]. She got to there ... She wanted to see how strong she can be because see, she always was a strong girl ...

    [Clare, age 65 with stomach cancer; Michael, age 67—husband; Anglo-Celtic]

Monitoring of appearance

Cosmetic status or physical appearance had a major impact on self-perception and powerfully reflected illness status to others. Good cosmesis facilitated the patient's caring for others and others' caring for the patient, as already seen with Monica *[Monica, age 48 with breast cancer; Alan, age late 50s—husband; Anglo-Celtic]* (see p. 35–6).

Monitoring the treatment type

Treatment status (for example, whether by morphine, chemotherapy, or radiotherapy) was an important lay marker of illness severity, and was also used to gauge progress:

MARIA ... the end is coming ... And because the chemotherapies have started, the last means of help have started, I think that ... whoever it may be, they will realise something in their minds [i.e. regarding the impending end]. As for me, I have taken it decisively. ...

    [Maria, age 69 with breast cancer; Peter, age 74—husband; Greek]

Monitoring via investigations

Medical investigations or tests were valuable progress markers for both doctors and families. However, tests sometimes inappropriately focused families on the concrete, measurable parameters of illness, thereby *reducing* it to a 'number on a piece of paper, or image on an X-ray film, or a colour change on a strip of paper' (Vafiadis, 1996). An example was seen in the family of a man who had chronic lymphocytic leukaemia, a mild form of leukaemia where patients usually survive for decades and often die of unrelated causes. The patient himself was well but his daughter unnecessarily agonised over his white blood cell counts:

ANASTASIA ... she is very super-anxious. She went and rang the Anti-Cancer Council and ... you know, went to the state library and looked in every book and [laughs] and [she'd say], "His neutrophils are low!", and you know ... it's not as if ... [it was critical] ... and [she'd] make sure that every time he goes [to hospital] they'd write down ... their results for *her* [emphasised] you know, ... But he's doing well ...   *[Anastasia, GP, age 31; Greek]*

Although favourable test results could dramatically raise hope, poor appreciation of their limitations could create lay confusion if a test failed to detect the underlying problem. Conversely, favourable test results could cause despair if the patient was sick, because the problem remained undefined and thus so did the chances for definitive help.

Monitoring according to response and progress

Response to treatment in terms of extent, rapidity, and duration, as well as the *temporal pattern* of progress, were important monitoring modalities. Poor response to treatment was often cited by Greek families to justify their concealment of information—the patient 'knew' anyway, without needing to be told. Conversely, good response to treatment or maintenance of a steady state sometimes engendered hope that was strong enough to overcome fear even when doctors expected deterioration:

PAULA ... the truth is ... because he had become well we weren't expecting him to become worse. ... With the ... radiotherapy that he had and everything stopped for quite a considerable period, and we thought that it had stopped ...
        [Aristotle, age 79 with prostate cancer; Paula, age ?—daughter; Greek]

Monitoring by comparison

Sometimes, monitoring was guided by comparison. Positive comparisons were common, where people compared their own situation to that of other cancer patients who were cured (or survived for a long time). This bolstered morale and could activate hope even in advanced illness:

DIMITRI ... in the beginning ... it wasn't so good ... and it wasn't so easy ... I knew other persons which had jumped over [i.e. overcome] this illness despite them being [very unwell—unclear words] ... I gave her courage and ... I told her about a certain uncle of mine, ... and he lived seventeen years. And in continuity we are now better off than what we were then with that knowledge; today, knowledge [or science] is advancing.

[Barbara, age 48 with cervical cancer; Dimitri, age 53—husband; Greek]

GPs also used positive comparisons as a strategy to help patients and families. Often, however, comparisons related by families were overwhelmingly negative:

PETER Well, as I see it with this, this illness, it passes ... as we see around us in the world, in five months, six months, each person [affected by it] succumbs.

[Maria, age 69 with breast cancer; Peter, age 74—husband; Greek]

Monitoring the actions and reactions of others

Clues about progress were also gleaned through the actions and reactions of others, including their subtle and non-verbal actions. Patients often monitored doctors in that way, but the doctors' views of the illness could also be affected by their own monitoring of the actions and reactions of patients and their families:

ANDREW ... he was actually quite an interesting person and ... once you got to know him he was really warm and friendly. He enjoyed it when I came around. ... He liked to talk. He'd get his wife to make me a coffee and a cake, you know. ... He would want to get all his sort of medical business out the way so we could sit down and have a little bit of a talk. ... I found that really, really good from my point of view. ...

[Andrew, GP, age early 40s; Greek]

Interaction with others was therefore important to the process of adjusting to transition. The following further examines this issue.

Adjustment to transition

Previous discussion on illness disclosure has already provided some background to the dynamics of adjustment. This process always took time:

PAULA To be truthful, he took it very, very badly in the beginning. He was worried ... I think now, not that he has overcome this, but he has gotten used to it. ... We always tell him that he will get well, he will get on, but he doesn't say that he will not, he doesn't say that he will. He ... understands that he cannot become any better.

[Aristotle, age 79 with prostate cancer; Paula, age ?—daughter; Greek]

Many families lived 'day by day' (for example, *[Aristotle, age 79 with prostate cancer; Paula, age ?—daughter; Greek]*), while others had definite plans in anticipation of future deterioration (as seen with *[Jane, English, age 61 with mycosis fungoides; John, German, age 70—husband]*, and *[Panteleimon, age 62 with lung cancer; Mary, age 63—wife; Greek]*). There seemed to be no strong link between acceptance of cancer and future planning. Few of those who accepted their poor prognosis spoke spontaneously and extensively about death itself, indicating that people often became 'used to it', rather than having 'overcome' it (as in the above quotation). This did not neatly fit Kubler-Ross' (1969) staged theory of acceptance because the attempt to normalise life was not denial (indeed, the devastating impact of diagnosis suggested acceptance, not denial). Rather, it was an attempt to view the illness in a balanced way without over-emphasising the negatives (see also Strauss, Corbin, Faberhaugh, Glaser, Maines et al., 1984 for further discussion on 'normalising', and Kellehear, 1990 for a critique of Kubler-Ross' theory of acceptance):

> **MICHAEL** ... how can I say it? We know it's there, we know everything there, but we don't talk about it ... incessantly, you know what I mean? ... It's there but, but it's not there to us ... That, that's how we're coping with it, put it that way. ... We know that's how it is.
>
> *[Clare, age 65 with stomach cancer; Michael, age 67—husband; Anglo-Celtic]*

GPs recognised that such responses were not denial, and did not insist on confronting people with the realities of the situation. They knew that a more complete and *contented* acceptance evolved as people psychologically *incorporated* the illness into their lives and identities. Such an incorporation made this phenomenon differ from Charmaz's (1990) notion of 'preferred identity', where people 'attempted to construct lives *apart* from the illness' (emphasis added). It was when illness was incorporated *into* one's life that various *gains* could be appreciated, even in advanced illness, and death could actively be prepared for:

> **MICHAEL** ... she doesn't ... look at the papers [now]. She used to always look at the papers. You know, she'd read it from go to whoa, she'd ... [read] everything that was in it. And, she used to love having a bet. ... That was her only vice, you know. Wasn't a vice—I didn't care, I mean ... she wasn't silly. She never spent any more than ... how much she could, you know what I mean? ... And ah, she loved to go to the races, you know, and ... well then she, as soon as she found out about this, ... she gave away her telephone betting. "Go on", it was eighty cents in it, I said, "Don't [close it]. Forget about it. Leave it". ... "Close it up, finish it", [she said]. Now ... that's

another part of her—everything ... is spot on. As soon as a bill comes—pay it. ... Even at this moment too, everything's gotta be, ... you know, finalised by her.

[Clare, age 65 with stomach cancer; Michael, age 67—husband; Anglo-Celtic]

Doctors often played an active role in guiding patients and families towards such a re-orientation. Byron *[Byron, GP, age 57; Anglo-Celtic]* likened it to '*training*' the family, noting that '*you've got to go through it all again*' when people unfamiliar to the situation stepped into it and disturbed its equilibrium. Doctors, however, also had to train themselves to adjust to transition, especially if they felt close to their patients:

ANASTASIA ... I actually worry about some of my patients now who are well, who are in their eighties who I'm attached to, 'cause I've been seeing them for two years ... and [they] have been well and I think, "Gosh you know in the next five years someone's gonna die", ... and ... that's probably worse off I reckon, in a way, 'cause a lot of the palliative patients, I've only known them as palliative patients. You know what I mean? *[Anastasia, GP, age 31; Greek]*

Site of care: the home versus the hospital

The need to examine situations in their unique context made the *site* of care an important topic. How did home-based care affect issues relating to control and power in interpersonal interaction? A study of the advantages and disadvantages of home care provided some clues.

Home-based care was beneficial in several ways. It enabled the patient and family to integrate their illness into normal, everyday life (Strauss et al., 1984). The very *presence* of the patient, even in end-stage illness, filled the need for companionship:

MARY ... When he was in hospital, then I couldn't [manage]. I saw the house as being a little empty; even if he is like this [i.e. in this state of advanced illness], I like it that he [is home] ... even if he is in bed; if he is alive [then it's OK] ... But if I came home from the hospital and saw this empty [house], I cried, I made a cup of coffee for myself alone, as it was ... I remained alone. I would go to my bed. Sometimes I would sleep, sometimes I wouldn't sleep. ... I would get up in the morning. The same—an empty house ... there was nothing to do. If you don't have a person [to look after], do you have chores?

[Panteleimon, age 62 with lung cancer; Mary, age 63—wife; Greek]

Home care enabled the family to support the patient, but also simultaneously *tested* their caring role. Advanced illness was emotionally challenging, but because there was little that anyone could offer the patient, apparently passive support tasks were paradoxically transformed into modes of very active, meaningful care (as already seen in the example of food provision, p. 80–1). The patient could also *monitor* and *care* for the family in a more *direct* way compared with the in-patient situation. The flexibility and lack of regimentation maximised such mutual support, in contrast to the hospital:

> **PAULA** ... the surrounds at home make him happy. At the hospital the setting doesn't make him happy. ... Because, let's say, they do their duty at the hospital; they will sit him in the chair—[if] they tell you that he will sit for one hour—*he will sit* [emphasised] for one hour. Just now I put him [on the chair], he had to sit for half an hour ... He couldn't. ... I was forced to put him back on the mattress.
>
> *[Aristotle, age 79 with prostate cancer; Paula, age ?—daughter; Greek]*

Home care also, however, held several disadvantages. Because the emotional domain belonged to the family, the visiting GP's sense of control was somewhat diminished, compared to the setting of their own surgery. This had practical ramifications. Byron *[Byron, GP, age 57; Anglo-Celtic]*, for example, noted that only basic medical equipment could be taken into the home, making him feel more vulnerable. The extra time that home-visits demanded was mentioned as an additional strain by only one of the GPs *[Margarita, GP, age 33; Greek]*, although after-hours work had universal ramifications for the GP's family:

> **CAROL** ... I was called out ... once in the middle of the night and once at around dinner time and [with] ... the 'around dinner time' one, ... I put the child in the car and brought him with me. ... And ah, that's obviously not very satisfactory ... I mean, he stayed in the car while I saw the patient, which didn't take very long. It turned out it wasn't a problem [that time], but you can't sort of say you're able to do things ... and then, you know, not be able to fulfil it. *[Carol, GP, age mid-30s; Anglo-Celtic]*

The home setting also took its toll on both patient and family. The often physically demanding tasks of care had to be balanced against other aspects of daily living, such as shopping, paying off bills, cleaning and going to work. Patients themselves, when able, actively engaged these non illness-related tasks, as seen with Monica *[Monica, age 48 with breast cancer; Alan, age late 50s—husband; Anglo-Celtic]* and Barbara *[Barbara, age 48 with cervical cancer; Dimitri, age 53—husband; Greek].* Residual time was thus scarce (Strauss et al., 1984).

The direct observation of the patient's deterioration was a major difficulty in home-based care. Decline did not have to be extensive to produce distress. Relative decline, such as subtle loss of a function that previously defined the patient's role and status, was as important as loss of more basic functions. Charles *[Charles, age 72 with prostate cancer; Amanda, age 72—wife; Anglo-Celtic]*, for example, a painter and plasterer by trade, struggled to accept initially that he could no longer do any painting around the house. Stress in the family also meant that the patient not only had to confront their own decline, but also the trauma on the family.

Home care also allowed the expression of *excessive support* (this was more limited in the hospital setting). Too much concern and too many visitors *physically exhausted* both patient and family, and also forced them to frequently *confront* emotional aspects of the illness that they might not wish to. Advanced or disfiguring illness also had the potential to distress visitors. It was this latter point, and a desire to maintain her own dignity, that dissuaded Clare *[Clare, age 65 with stomach cancer; Michael, age 67—husband; Anglo-Celtic]* from receiving visitors.

Although families acquired medical skills through home care (such as urinary catheter management, giving injections, skin care, bowel management, symptom monitoring, and others), difficult symptoms sometimes made home care inferior to being in the hospital. The home was not equipped to manage unexpected and frightening emergencies, such as acute epilepsy, haematemesis, sudden dyspnoea, and others.

Financial difficulties with home care occupied only a small place in the interviews, and these mainly related to the medication costs (as seen with *[Barbara, age 48 with cervical cancer; Dimitri, age 53—husband; Greek]*). Hospital-type beds, oxygen, and other equipment were supplied through the hospice services.

Although no culture or gender-specific issues favouring or not favouring the home were apparent, anecdotal hospice experience suggested that these affected *how* home care was provided. The Southport Hospice, for instance, often bathed Greek females but only rarely Greek males, because, culturally, that was the wife's responsibility. *'One of the few Greek men we washed' [Abbreviated field notes; conversation with director of Southport Hospice]* had suffered a stroke and his wife had severe osteoarthritis.

Generally, a certain optimal mix of conditions were needed for successful home care. These related to the illness type and its amenability to such care, time and resource availability, and family dynamics. Efficient symptom control relied on a composed medical presence to guide the process of dying. Ultimately, however, as one GP put it:

> **ANASTASIA** ... to some people dying at home is still a new concept, it's a new fad and ... you've got to, I think, probably pick the right family to do that for.
>
> *[Anastasia, GP, age 31; Greek]*.

Interaction, change and uncertainty: summary and implications for medical power

Having examined the meeting of medical and lay worlds during critical periods in cancer illness, reflection is now made on how this analysis informs the study of medical power itself. This task is encapsulated by the following three key questions, relating to what form medical power took, where it was socially located, and how it was expressed.

What form does medical power take?

This proved a difficult question because medical power was not an absolute and concrete phenomenon, but was instead highly dependent on the specific illness context. Medical power could thus be expressed and manifested in a variety of ways, relating to either the doctor's medical knowledge, their technical expertise or skill, their social standing, their devotion to the patient, their availability, their emotional composure, their confidence, their manner of dress, their specific use of their title of 'Doctor', and even their ability to concede power by admitting and accepting their own limitations.

Medical power, therefore, was never *total* but instead *selective*: control and strength could be exhibited in certain areas while shortcomings were apparent in others. Shortcomings, by definition, were universal in palliative care, because the illness was not curable. The selective nature of medical power, however, did not necessarily diminish the overall standing of the doctor in the eyes of the patient. Recall, for example, Jane's *[Jane, English, age 61 with mycosis fungoides; John, German, age 70—husband]* admiration of her dermatologist, a highly competent doctor who was interested in her in an academic rather than a personal way.

Medical power was thus potentially *paradoxical*. It could be present when it seemingly should not be, as seen in the relationship between

Andrew *[Andrew, GP, age early 40s; Greek]* and his patient with prostate cancer, where closeness and mutual admiration progressively strengthened *as the patient deteriorated.* Conversely, medical power could be absent when it seemingly should be present, as seen with Anastasia's *[Anastasia, GP, age 31; Greek]* patient with controlled chronic lymphocytic leukaemia. In this latter instance, the relatively benign nature of the illness could not allay the concerns of the patient's daughter, who was perhaps reacting to the *name* of the illness more than to its immediate threat.

The paradoxical nature of medical power leads to a consideration of the next major question about it—where, in fact, is medical power socially and personally located?

Where is medical power located?

The Introduction pointed out that there is still a general respect for medicine's ability and authority, despite criticism of it being too distant and scientific. Power was therefore socially located within the *discipline of medicine* itself. However, this power also made medicine more accountable, leading to more person-centred, rather than disease-centred, approaches. It also contributed to the modern phenomenon of medical litigation, showing that the general recognition given to medicine is *not* automatically conveyed to the individual doctor. Rather, the individual doctor has to continually live up to the generally high standing of medicine. Medical power, therefore, was also located within the *individual doctor*, provided they were competent enough to possess and utilise it. The narratives of both GPs, patients and carers showed that the doctor often had to prove themselves in some way, usually in knowledge, caring, interest, or skill. Sometimes, they were directly confronted to do so, as in the scenarios of role-forcing that have been described. At other times, the doctor was tested in a more furtive manner, such as being required to demonstrate their ability with a decoy problem before being entrusted with the real problem. An example related to Anastasia *[Anastasia, GP, age 31; Greek]* who was initially presented with diabetes before the new patient entrusted her with his diagnosis of Burkitt's lymphoma.

The corollary to the need of the individual doctor to demonstrate competence and to wield their medical power was that they had to be *allowed* to do so. This was only possible if the patient and family recognised such actions as constituting power. Comprehensive medical knowledge, for example, that was insensitive was of little avail to patients and families who valued a more personal and caring approach above all else. In such a scenario, medical knowledge, the supposed cornerstone of medical power, could be transformed into, or interpreted as, medical bullying, dominance or dismissiveness. An example related to the situation of Paraskevi and her family *[Paraskevi, age 48 with cervical cancer; Mark, age 23—son; Greek]*, who felt completely abandoned when they were frankly told of her diagnosis of incurable cervical cancer and the limited therapeutic options available. This indicates that *patients and families themselves* constituted a key location of medical power, because they ultimately ratified it and gave it validity at the individual level.

The unpredictability of cancer illness, however, also suggested that determinants of medical power were also located *beyond* the individual persons of the doctor, the patient or the carer, and beyond the general social perceptions of the body of medicine as a whole. In this sense, medical power was elusive and to a certain degree determined by circumstances generated through pure *chance*. This was illustrated in the fortuitous circumstances for the calming of Carol's psychotic patient *[Carol, GP, age mid-30s; Anglo-Celtic]* (see p. 80).

Although chance could be entirely fortuitous, it could also be more calculated, as in medical risk-taking. Risks had to be taken in diagnosis, regarding the relevance of given symptoms and how far it was appropriate to pursue them. Similarly, risks also had to be taken in treatment, especially cancer treatment, where many forms of therapy were in themselves life-threatening.

Outcomes, however, could also be negative even in situations where they were not expected to be, that is, in situations where risk was absolutely minimal. Anastasia *[Anastasia, GP, age 31; Greek]*, for instance, related the event of administering influenza vaccine to her healthy mother. Her mother had a rare but severe local reaction to the vaccine, shaking Anastasia's sense of control and reinforcing her previous hunch that doctors should not provide medical care for their relatives.

Outcomes could also be unexpectedly positive. These could resurrect a sense of medical control and power that might otherwise have been flagging. For example, Brendan's *[Brendan, age mid-40s with cerebral glioma; Michelle, age ?—wife]* unexpected survival of multiple cancer diagnoses in the past raised hopes of the ability of the doctors to emulate the same feat (i.e. cure) in him again.

In summary, then, medical power was not only socially located within the *discipline of medicine*, but to varying degrees also resided in the *individual doctor* themselves, in *patients and families*, and in the uncontrollable realm of *chance* itself.

How is medical power expressed?

Pre-existing notions of medical power in both doctor and patient were ultimately expressed and refined in each situation through interpersonal interaction. Medical power was *relative*, that is, dependent on interpretations of concrete medical actions rather than on their absolute level of 'medical correctness'. Interaction re-moulded original conceptions of medical power held by both doctor and patient. Such interaction was not a static phenomenon—it progressed through *time*. Medical power could therefore *fluctuate* over time according to how continually changing illness circumstances and emotions were negotiated.

Although the ideal goal of all participants was always a harmony between doctor, patient and family, such harmony was sometimes elusive. If the unique perspective of the single individual was challenging enough to the establishment of harmony, then what of the interaction between *multiple persons,* who viewed the illness from different 'angles'? This would seem to place harmony and compatibility even further out of reach. The implications for the multidisciplinary nature of palliative care are considerable. Attention therefore needs to be turned towards summarising the essential prerequisites for harmony in interaction.

Prerequisites for doctor–patient harmony: an insight into the nature of medical power

Harmony and compatibility were crucial for both defining and sustaining medical power. Although medical power could exist and be expressed in a disharmonious state, such 'power' was short lived, cutting off its own expression, because dissonance destroyed the doctor–patient relationship. An example was seen with the surgeon who wanted to give Monica *[Monica, age 48 with breast cancer; Alan, age late 50s—husband; Anglo-Celtic]* a radical mastectomy, against the feelings of the oncologist and Monica herself. Compatibility between the views of doctor, patient and carer, on the other hand, reinforced the doctor's standing and also conferred a sense of control (and therefore power) to patients and their families.

The interaction between medical and non-medical worlds has been shown to be dynamically complex. It is emotionally fragile, involves a multiplicity of persons, and is subject to swift, undesirable and often unexpected changes, in keeping with the typically rapid evolution of cancer illness. Despite this, however, compatibility between all parties was neither out of reach nor rare, provided that four major conditions were satisfied (see Box 2.3).

BOX 2.3 Key prerequisites for doctor–patient harmony

---

1 A consistency of views and approaches towards illness **within** medical and non-medical worlds, respectively.

2 A mutual realisation that existing therapeutic frameworks, both medical and lay, are **relative** and not absolute.

3 A need for medical and non-medical worlds to **support** each other by being sensitive to how each views and experiences the illness.

4 A need to realise the first three prerequisites **early** in the illness, before relationships become irrevocably damaged.

First, there had to be compatibility of views *within* the non-medical and medical worlds, respectively, before there could be any real chance of harmony *between* them. Several examples were raised of disagreement within families about the aims and progress of treatment, which effectively paralysed medical power because of the doubts that were raised. Sometimes that caused role-forcing (Glaser & Strauss, 1965), or the complete abandonment of the medical team in preference for a new one (which further delayed and complicated treatment because of the time involved in the familiarisation process). Conversely, incompatibility could exist within the medical and allied health professions regarding the approach to a particular clinical situation, with equally destructive effects. Examples were provided regarding disclosure and the choice of treatment regimen. Although such different emphases were in themselves not 'wrong' in an absolute sense, they were not appropriately *explained or applied* to the particular clinical situation.

The second prerequisite for compatibility between medical and non-medical worlds was a mutual realisation that the existing frameworks, both medical and lay, for approaching the management of illness were *not absolute*; concrete rules were *absent*. In the case of the medical profession, the clinical approach had to be *constructed* using pre-existing therapeutic frameworks only as a *guideline*, rather than as 'solid' structures that were assumed to represent the 'truth' and 'reality'. Examples of this phenomenon were seen in the issue of disclosure, where GPs effectively used uncertainty to minimise the pain of an unfavourable disclosure, or graded disclosure over time, or tried to balance negative aspects in disclosure with positive aspects.

However, because pre-existing moral frameworks in both patient and practitioner were often quite solid or rigid, the flexibility required to *construct* a clinical approach (as opposed to *applying* it) was often limited. With disclosure, for instance, doctors, under family pressure not to disclose a diagnosis, were not prepared to lie to the patient or to conceal the truth if directly asked about it. Additionally, the attractiveness of a certain, concrete approach, itself so appealing to scientific thinking, sometimes saw doctors revert to using pre-existing therapeutic frameworks as rules rather than guidelines, often with negative consequences (recall, for example, Margarita's *[Margarita, GP, age 33; Greek]* frustration if her patients did not adopt healthy diets).

The power of the rational, sure, scientific approach was not confined to the medical profession but also permeated into patient and carer thought, generating problems. A striking example was the perplexity generated in families when 'high-tech' medical tests failed to diagnose their disease. Tests were seen as precise and definitive tools rather than mere guides in the diagnostic or monitoring process.

The third pre-requisite for compatibility between medical and non-medical worlds was the ability of each to read how the other was viewing and experiencing the illness. This depended not only upon individual personalities but also on the structure of the health-care system, which determined consultation time-frames, accessibility and health-care costs. Compatibility between doctor, patient and family was enhanced not only through such *mutual understanding*, but through the opportunities it raised for *mutual support*. Medical awareness, for example, of the impact of symptoms upon families heightened the GP's appreciation of problems that might otherwise have seemed trivial; 'passive' symptomatic treatment then became 'active' treatment, and when viewed in that light could strengthen medical enthusiasm and zeal. Medical control was then possible even in very negative illness situations, either through the persistence of the medical presence itself, or by its reflection on positive aspects, or by using uncertainty itself as a clinically advantageous tool.

Patients and families themselves also supported their doctors through their realisation that the medical task was often difficult and that doctors themselves could not work miracles. Mutual understanding therefore paradoxically transformed difficulties into benefits because the *mutual appreciation* of the predicament of the other often became a self-perpetuating process throughout the illness.

The fourth prerequisite was that the first three prerequisites had to be realised *early* in the illness before irrevocable damage to the doctor–patient relationship had been done. Unfavourable events early in the illness reverberated strongly in the minds of patient and carer throughout all of its subsequent phases, *irrespective* of how well handled the latter were. This was powerfully expressed in the narratives of Maria and Peter *[Maria, age 69 with breast cancer; Peter, age 74—husband; Greek]*, Monica *[Monica, age 48 with breast cancer; Alan, age late 50s—husband; Anglo-Celtic]*, and Panteleimon and Mary *[Panteleimon, age 62 with lung cancer; Mary, age 63—wife; Greek]*, where major traumas in diagnosis still persisted. Conversely, favourable events and progress early in the illness had the opposite effect, and could actually dull the impact of subsequent negative experiences, as seen with the illnesses of Charles *[Charles, age 72 with prostate cancer; Amanda, age 72—wife; Anglo-Celtic]*, Barbara *[Barbara, age 48 with cervical cancer; Dimitri, age 53—husband; Greek]*, and Simon *[Simon, age 64 with lymphoma; Cynthia, age 52—wife; Anglo-Celtic]*. Circumstances therefore had to be optimised early, which was difficult because that period of the illness was one of its most emotionally intense and confronting periods. It was also a time where the doctor and patient were *least* familiar with each other. That was so even if a pre-existing and longstanding GP-patient relationship had existed prior to the intrusion of cancer. The explanation for this lay in the fact that cancer, being a serious illness and necessitating more intense contact and support, tested and revealed *new* aspects of the personality of the doctor and the patient, both to themselves as well as to each other.

Conclusion: the effects of uncertainty on doctor–patient compatibility

Illness circumstances could not always be adequately controlled, predicted, nor objectively 'worked through', because of the problem of *uncertainty* (Strauss et al., 1984). Uncertainty was present in the illness experience of every patient, carer and GP. It was a universal phenomenon that formed the major barrier to compatibility between medical and non-medical worlds in cancer illness, having the ability to tarnish each of the four prerequisites for doctor–patient/carer harmony that have just been discussed.

Uncertainty could relate to the medical condition of the cancer, such as its optimal treatment, its response to treatment, and its likely future progress. However, dilemmas were usually not purely medical, but had extensive *moral, ethical* and *medico-legal* implications. For example, should treatment be initiated, continued or stopped? When, and at whose discretion? There, in particular, the openness of the patient-centred method could *generate* uncertainty if patient and family wishes extended beyond the finite boundaries of GP flexibility (or vice versa). Uncertainty was also inherent in *how* one interacted with others. Some examples related to *what* was communicated to others and *how* that was done, and *which emotions* were openly shown versus which remained hidden. Further still, uncertainty also had an existential component that related to the religious and philosophical issues of how physical death would affect personal existence and being.

A formal study of the enigma of uncertainty therefore becomes necessary for a more complete understanding of the nature of medical power and how it influences compatibility between the world of the doctor and the world of the patient and carer. The following chapter introduces and examines the concept of medical uncertainty and its implications on doctor–patient harmony and medical power.

3

The challenge of medical uncertainty

Chapter 2 has shown that the interaction between doctor and patient was crucial in shaping the form and ultimate expression of medical power. The common stereotype of such an expression, where the doctor rigidly and impersonally controlled the relationship, was uncommon. Such an approach was often not welcomed by doctors, patients and families alike, and its presence fractured relationships and thereby stifled its own existence.

It was harmony and compatibility between all parties that enhanced medicine's status and hence its power. Medical power was therefore paradoxically greatest when it yielded some of its control to the patient and family in accordance with the principles of the patient-centred approach. However, medical power was sometimes expected to be (and had to be) dominant and directive according to its own medical expertise and judgment, *without* sacrificing patient centredness (Silverman, 1987; Maseide, 1991). The resulting confidence that such directive approaches imparted to families actually *facilitated* the patient-centred approach.

The harmony, however, that was so vital to the therapeutic relationship was continually threatened by uncertainty. Little about cancer could be certain, whether this related to diagnostic aspects such as its presence or absence, its likely course in a given individual, the best therapeutic options for it, or its personal effects on people.

This chapter examines medical uncertainty (that is, the uncertainty faced by GPs) in cancer care and its impact on the clinical relationship. It begins by describing different *types* of uncertainty (see Box 3.1) and their consequences. A theoretical overview of the issue of uncertainty follows, and conclusions are drawn regarding its effect upon doctor–patient harmony and medical authority. Throughout the chapter, patient and carer uncertainties are incorporated and considered because they actively contributed to medical uncertainty, and were in turn profoundly affected by it. Medical uncertainty, therefore, does not only refer to an uncertainty *intrinsic* to doctors (as Fox, 1957 suggests), but also to an uncertainty that is generated from their interaction with patients and their families, and by the nature of cancer illness itself.

BOX 3.1 Major categories of medical uncertainty

Knowledge-related uncertainty   Uncertainty in the individual doctor
Uncertainty within the profession as a whole
Uncertainty in the individual or in the profession?

Uncertainty related to health-care structure

Process-related uncertainty   Interpersonal uncertainty
The limitations of language
Ambiguity in the location of responsibility
Technical uncertainty

Inherent medical uncertainty   Inherent uncertainty in the nature of illness and
its treatment
Existential uncertainty

Uncertainty in the negotiation of different paradigms of illness

---

Moral and emotional uncertainty

Knowledge-related uncertainty

The fallacious belief that medical process was made *routine* and *controllable* (see the Introduction) was a legacy of the scientific revolution in medicine. Although the patient-centred approach amended the purely biological view of the human person, it has not significantly altered the view of medicine as a rigidly controllable process. Foucault (1994: 97) noted that in the latter part of the eighteenth century, 'medicine discovered that uncertainty may be treated, analytically, as the sum of a certain number of isolatable degrees of certainty that were capable of rigorous calculation'.

Medical uncertainty is therefore often discussed as an issue of *knowledge*, rather than as an issue of *process* or *interaction* or *limitation*.

Fox (1957) exemplified this view in her study of clinical uncertainty in cohorts of medical students at differing levels of seniority. Although Fox's (1957) underemphasis of *certainty* in medicine and her narrow focus on knowledge alone as the core issue in uncertainty have drawn criticism (see Atkinson, 1984), her three knowledge-based classes of uncertainty merit discussion.

Uncertainty in the individual doctor

The vastness of medicine by definition meant that uncertainty in the individual doctor was inevitable: 'No one can have at his [sic] command all skills and all knowledge of the lore of medicine' (Fox, 1957: 208). Such uncertainty was commonly present in the GP* informants, but did not seem difficult to overcome. Many sought guidance from specialists, colleagues, and books held in the surgery, or did personal homework to research their uncertainty. Most of the GPs had no difficulty in sharing this type of uncertainty with their patients:

> **ELIZABETH** ... And I feel that ... particularly with the young patients these days, .. they don't perceive the doctor to be ... the almighty who ... knows everything, 'cause we don't. I mean ... sometimes I have to go out and look things up ... and I let them know that, I say, "Look, I'm not sure about a particular issue, and ... do you mind if I just look it up and I, I'll let you know?" ...   *[Elizabeth, GP, age 32; Croatian]*

Patients also, both Greek and Anglo–Celtic, were generally comfortable in accepting these limitations. However, they also needed to feel that the doctor would address such uncertainty in a responsible manner, be that looking up textbooks, seeking the advice of colleagues, or by some other means. Further, such action had to be appropriately *timed* according to the problem's perceived level of severity.

Uncertainty within the profession as a whole

Many clinical problems exceeded the bounds of current medical knowledge: 'There are innumerable questions to which no physician, however well trained, can as yet provide answers' (Fox, 1957: 208). This type of uncertainty was commonly experienced by medical specialists and GPs involved in palliative care. GPs in particular, especially if the patient chose to die at home, were vividly confronted by the powerlessness and uncertainty of medicine over the process of death. One GP referred to it as a sombre and *'humbling experience' [Frank, GP, age early 30s; Anglo-Celtic]*. Specialists were also affected, in sharp contrast to views (Fox, 1957; Light, 1979) that specialisation in a narrower field was a means of mastering or limiting uncertainty. For example, many forms of chemotherapy initiated by specialists were located at the boundaries of existing medical knowledge. Tumours not responding to conventional therapy, or tumours with no definitive protocol for their management, forced 'best-guess' therapeutic approaches.

Patients and families coped with this type of uncertainty in varying ways. Monica *[Monica, age 48 with breast cancer; Alan, age late 50s—husband; Anglo-Celtic]* and her family were greatly comforted by the meticulous approach of their medical oncologist, conveying a sense that everything possible was being done to select the best treatment option. Acceptance of the ultimate biological finitude of life also assisted people in coming to terms with this type of medical uncertainty.

In cases of poor prognosis, general uncertainty within the body of medicine was more acceptable than uncertainty that resided in an individual doctor, because the former was not as avoidable, and therefore engendered less sense of loss. Maria *[Maria, age 69 with breast cancer; Peter, age 74—husband; Greek]*, for example, readily accepted the inability of medicine to cure her, but there was still a conviction that the original GP had been personally at fault for failing to diagnose cancer as the cause of her protracted prodromal symptoms.

Uncertainty in the individual or in the profession?

This category of medical uncertainty was related to the previous two. Here, there 'was difficulty in distinguishing between personal ignorance or ineptitude and the limitations of present medical knowledge' (Fox, 1957: 208–9). Fox (1957), for example, noted that subtle physical signs, such as a soft cardiac murmur, could be diagnostically challenging even to experienced auscultators. In such cases, students or inexperienced doctors were more likely to attribute their difficulty in clinical diagnosis to personal inability, rather than realising, as did experienced clinicians, that the physical signs were challenging and not straightforward.

The rapid advances in diagnostic and treatment modalities for cancer made this category relevant to the GP informants, because the challenge to keep up to date was great. This challenge made them question whether their uncertainty stemmed from themselves or was endemic to the body of medical science as a whole.

The problem, however, was not only linked with the doctors' need to keep up to date. A more subtle side effect of the revolution in medical knowledge has been the *creation* of uncertainty itself. The Introduction mentioned the progressive shifts in diagnosis towards earlier and earlier phases of illness through the use of scientific understanding and technology. That process alone, and the accompanying shifts in public and medical expectation, caused dilemmas in many areas of practice. The current thinking about bowel cancer, for instance, notes that any change in bowel habit may herald the condition (Kumar & Clark, 1994). However, the expensive and invasive means of adequate investigation (usually colonoscopy or barium enema), together with the obscurity of what a 'significant change in bowel habit' actually means (especially towards the more minor range of the symptom spectrum), can create considerable medical confusion. Similarly, taking the example of Fox (1957) regarding diagnostic uncertainty in cardiac auscultation, it was only after the stethoscope was advanced enough to detect subtle cardiac sounds and murmurs that this category of knowledge-based uncertainty was created.

Further than this, scientific advances introduced non-knowledge-related categories of uncertainty into clinical practice. The artificial ventilator is an example. After its invention, a host of moral issues sprang up that did not previously exist, such as who should have priority access to it, the duration of its use, and the difficult issue of when or if it should ever be turned off, and by whom.

Implications of knowledge–related uncertainty

All categories of knowledge-related uncertainty were not free-standing but were instead linked to, and affected by, further tiers of complexity. First, they could actually be *generated* by advances in knowledge, as already outlined. Second, they also led to different forms of uncertainty, relating more to ethics and morals than to scientific knowledge itself. Third, a major challenge to doctors was *how* their knowledge-based uncertainty and all of its subsequent ramifications was actually shared with patient and family (that is, what was shared, with whom, and when). The section on disclosures in Chapter 2 revealed the nature of this complexity.

The relevant conclusion here, in agreement with Light (1979), Young (1981), and Atkinson (1984), is that there is much more to medical uncertainty than limitations in medical knowledge alone. In particular, 'medical knowledge needs to be viewed in terms of the processes by which it is produced, rather than in terms of its structure. ... When processual and structural views of medical knowledge are compared, the latter are found to either bracket out important emotional and ideological determinants, or to trivialise them' (Young, 1981). Fox's (1957) own data is rich in such 'processual' determinants, but as Atkinson (1984) and Light (1979) have correctly noted, these are not incorporated into her summation of the problem of medical uncertainty.

The view of the clinical process as a sequential, 'unfolding event' (Fisher, 1984) sees earlier events, often not purely related to issues of medical knowledge, determine the nature of subsequent ones. This broadens the problem of medical uncertainty beyond the issue of knowledge alone (see also Katz, 1985 for practical examples relating to surgical practice). The following sections examine these areas of uncertainty in more detail.

Uncertainty related to health-care structure

Uncertainty was not only located in knowledge but also in *setting* and in *conflicts of setting*. The latter was especially important for GPs, who are caught between two very different worlds, to which they simultaneously belong and between which they continually mediate (Rosser & Maguire, 1982). One of these worlds is that of technological biomedicine, represented by the tertiary hospital. This institution is instrumental in the GP's own training and oriented towards curing illness. The other world is the GP's actual community, where the impacts of illness are felt and lived, and which is more oriented to the notion of healing. Concomitant belonging to these conflicting realms creates pressures on the GP, and this, rather than lack of knowledge, might explain shortfalls observed in their cancer management (Rosser & Maguire, 1982).

The conflicting demands of these two realms caused GP uncertainty because many divergent issues had to be considered. These ranged from likelihood of serious illness, potential impacts of different courses of action, time constraints in general practice, consequences of action versus inaction; and availability, ease and cost of external diagnostic and treatment resources. Such difficulty was illustrated by Ben *[Ben, GP, age 49; Jewish]*, a GP who attended a patient with end-stage brain cancer when their regular GP was away for the day. The patient was on dexamethasone, a drug that had effectively reduced swelling around the brain tumour, but which also produced a very high blood sugar level:

> **BEN** ... I asked one of the other staff about what ... he'd recommend and it was an immediate admission [to hospital] and ... I spent half the day contacting [Dr. E, the regular GP] and I got a very strong order, "Bugger off!" ... And ... [he] then took the reins, ... [and] exercised the ... necessary control and care. It's not always easy, I mean obviously it can be very, very extending but ... there was a lesson in that one, I tell you. *[Ben, GP, age 49; Jewish]*

The 'lesson' for Ben was that although his hospital training suggested that hospital admission was the most definitive way of management, it would be ... :

> **BEN** ... very irritating for a primary care giver to find that their patient ... has ended up in a hospital because they've got a high blood sugar, when in fact that person is clearly dying and it really isn't hardly the point any more, and that they would prefer that they stayed at home with support of ... family around them, and that they'd set up this process [for] God knows how long.
> *[Ben, GP, age 49; Jewish].*

The patient died peacefully at home a week or so later, making the decision to maintain home care the 'correct' one. However, even with the best of planning, unexpected circumstances might easily have made such a decision the 'wrong' one. For instance, the patient might have exsanguinated at home after a massive haematemesis secondary to dexamethasone-induced peptic ulceration. Pros and cons were weighed up, however, and a calculated clinical *risk* was taken that then steered the management in a particular direction. Difficulties would be created, however, if 'a nameless lawyer warned a faceless bureaucrat that a risk existed' (Mitchell, 1997). Such risk-taking was a part of the practical reality of medicine, especially of everyday general practice. Theodore's *[Theodore, GP, age 63; Greek]* comments about the management of febrile children without an obvious focus also highlighted this point:

> **THEODORE** ... if I have the slightest doubt they get referred. ... I've never hesitated about that. ... But occasionally ... you can't refer them because, well, a kid with a temperature of 40 degrees, [a] one year old child, I mean you can't just

refer everybody, a child with 40 degrees ... and you sweat a little bit on that. ...
But in general if something's funny or ... it's a gut reaction, if you don't like what
[you see] ... you refer them ...   [Theodore, GP, age 63; Greek]

The hospital laboratory could perform a septic work-up on a febrile child and exclude a potentially life-threatening illness, such as bacterial meningitis. However, the commonness of fever without an obvious focus in young children, the rarity of acute bacterial meningitis, the trauma of a septic work-up for child and parents, and the chaos on available resources that would be caused if every such child were referred, all pointed to the acceptability of a conservative approach.

Many similar situations were described in cancer illness, often relating to the question of whether symptoms represented a recurrence or a progression of disease. They sometimes also concerned more practical issues. Byron [Byron, GP, age 57; Anglo-Celtic], for example, noted the difficulties in organising pathology services to visit the patient's home. He also described the practical limitations of the home visit, in that it separated the doctor from the diagnostic and management facilities located in their clinic.

Implications of uncertainty related to health-care structure

The pressures and conflicts generated by the health-care structure and setting were considerable. In their own right, they could be far more important sources of GP uncertainty than a lack of medical knowledge alone. Often, however, these processes were harder to appreciate and understand from a purely theoretical (or 'outsider') perspective. Although patients and carers often had good insight into the dilemmas and the calculated risk-taking inherent in clinical practice, such insight was not universal. In these instances, it seemed harder to bridge the distance that this created between the GP and the family compared to distance caused by a lack of knowledge. This was because issues related to health-care structure were often more subtle and complex. The same was also found for uncertainties relating to medical process, which will now be considered.

Process-related uncertainty

Uncertainty, located both in medical knowledge and in the social and health-care structure, was also manifestly present in the face to face *process* of the medical encounter. Light (1979) breaks up this process into its *temporal* sequence, and coins distinct categories of uncertainty relating to both diagnosis and treatment. However, at their root, Light's (1979) process-related categories of uncertainty all share and are all underpinned by several key interactional points that are described below.

Interpersonal uncertainty

As discussed, the structural emphasis proposed by Rosser and Maguire (1982) about GP uncertainty in cancer care focused excessively on *conflict* or *confusion* between the realms of disease (as defined by scientific biomedicine) and illness (as defined by the patient and family). Although important, it tended to negate the weight of inherent human emotion present within *any* given context, and assumed uniform and distinct conceptions of disease and illness across society. Equally important, therefore, were the *actual* stresses associated *with* and *within* each framework (that is, the curing biomedical-hospital framework versus the healing folk-community framework), in addition to the differences between them.

Still and Todd (1986) went some way towards addressing this issue by theorising about differing frameworks of operation at the level of the *illness itself*, rather than at the *structural level* of Rosser and Maguire (1982). Still and Todd hypothesised the existence of specific GP 'roles' to parallel differing patient roles, concluding that a hypothetical doctor *'ideal type'* (a so-called *'caring role'*) that corresponded to the patient's dying role was still *evolving*, and distinct from the conventional *'curative role'* that paralleled patients' sick roles (Still & Todd, 1986). This was a proposed focus of uncertainty, although the concept is plagued by two major problems. First, the unique and complex nature of an individual's emotions raises questions as to whether the notion of a *generalised* medical 'ideal type' in palliative care is a valid concept at all. Second, the proposition that the ideal caring type is *still evolving* is challenged at the individual level by the abundance of close and caring GP–patient–family relationships observed in this study. Further, such good relationships were not unusual between patients and hospital specialists (who are often unjustly presumed to be too scientific and less patient-centred). Even doctors who fulfilled the 'caring role' of Still and Todd (1986) at the individual level still had difficulties in dealing with grey areas and other stressful aspects in the process of care. Therefore, although medical uncertainty could be tempered to a degree by moulding the medical role to the patient's dying role, it could not be eliminated, because the ideal 'caring role' was neither uniform nor stress-free, and therefore it was not without uncertainty.

One source of such uncertainty was the unpredictability of patient or family response to particular illness events, including their level of cooperation with the doctor and the type of compromise and negotiation that might be needed as a result. Light (1979) called this type of uncertainty the 'uncertainty of client response', and Chapter 2 provided many examples of it.

For the GP, parallels to 'uncertainty of client response' extended to medical specialists to produce 'uncertainty of specialist colleague response'. Interpersonal uncertainty in their interactions with specialist colleagues could create considerable tension in GPs. GP discomfort at appearing incompetent in the eyes of the specialist was a powerful phenomenon, and even applied to specialists with whom the GP had a *good* relationship:

> MARGARITA ... if [my GP colleagues are not available for another opinion], or they're not sure, ... I ring up a specialist ...and ... I've got a few specialists that I'm more comfortable with ... and ... they're really good. ... They'll speak with me ... quite easily and freely and ... I've got some who are *really, really* [emphasis] good and you know, they, they don't make fun of me [giggles] or anything. I'll ask a really basic question and they'll say, "Yeah, no problems". [Both Margarita and the interviewer laugh]. And I think that that's *really* [emphasised] important with being able to ... communicate well with the specialists. ...
>
> *[Margarita, GP, age 33; Greek]*

The notion of a medical hierarchy therefore exerted its own unique influence within the medical profession. Medical power not only emanated from doctors but also acted upon them through the persons of their colleagues. (The study's scope was too limited to assess whether uncertainty and anxiety about colleague response also applied to the medical specialist in their dealings with GPs—this area awaits further research.)

The limitations of language

Another process-related category of uncertainty stemmed from limitations in the process of communication. Language had a limited ability to express innermost feelings and to convey knowledge. This limitation was *not* exclusively related to the many practical constraints that challenged effective doctor–patient communication (examples of these are the need to maintain hope, which affected the nature and topic of communication; the time constraints on consultations; or the threat of medico-legal reprisal, which favours defensive medicine and thus formalises clinical interaction). Rather, language itself held important inherent limitations in its expressive ability that were *independent* of these practical constraints against it.

The way that the doctor's explanation of the clinical problem was interpreted by the patient or family depended on their perceptions of the situation. Panteleimon *[Panteleimon, age 62 with lung cancer; Mary, age 63— wife; Greek]*, for example, was devastated by his diagnosis because of his fear of cancer, even though there were active therapies available at the time of diagnosis.

Likewise, the way patients and families viewed and reported their symptoms determined how effectively the doctor *interpreted* that information, *independent* of the doctor's clinical knowledge. Ultimately, for the doctor, symptomatology had to be reconstituted into a biomedical format (reflecting their medical training and justifying the management plan) that was in the English language (for the purposes of medical note-taking and communication with medical colleagues). Symptoms, however, could be presented in ways that were not conducive to such re-interpretation (Light, 1979):

> **MATTHEW** ... I find it harder sometimes to ... separate out what's important, and what's not important ... You ... get an ... idea of some symptoms, you know "Well, I'd like that fixed", but it's not obviously that important, or urgent, and then ... you get the view of which ones are really important, but [with] Greeks, sort of almost everything is equally 'un-pressing' [some emphasis here] ... and that sometimes means you ... have to sort through ... ten different things to see ... if there's anything that is significant. ... And I don't know if I'm the only one who finds that, but, because you just get presented with a whole lot of complaints, and you either have to deal with each one totally and separately or ... treat every one with a ... with equal triviality, or ... or whatever ... Do you find that? ...
>
> *[Matthew, GP, age mid-30s; Greek]*

GP strategies to bridge the diagnostic distance in such circumstances were either to down-play emphasis given to some symptoms or else assess them all. Both situations could delay diagnosis (Figure 3.1).

That Greek descriptions and interpretations of symptoms proved difficult for a Greek GP like Matthew *[Matthew, GP, age mid-30s; Greek]* showed that

FIGURE 3.1 Models for diagnostic delay

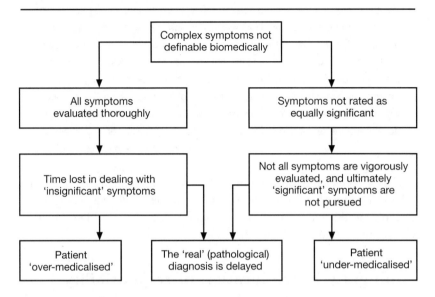

cultural compatibility did *not* assure doctor–patient harmony. This was *contrary* to suggestions by an Australian conference on multicultural health (Southern Sydney Area Health Service, 1993). Nor was a shared language sufficient to provide a clear interpretation of meaning:

> **MATTHEW** ... I'm not sure whether the symptoms and the language ... even with Greek doctors ...
> **INTERVIEWER** Whether they carry the equivalent weight ...
> **MATTHEW** Mmm [in agreement]. ... There's a concern that in lots of symptoms, like the same words don't mean the same things.
> *[Matthew, GP, age mid-30s; Greek]*

Meaning, of course, was not restricted to the pathology of the illness, but applied to emotions associated with it. Carol's *[Carol, GP, age mid-30s; Anglo-Celtic]* difficulty in expressing her emotions to her husband, the person closest to her, illustrated this point:

> **CAROL** ... sometimes its something that happens in there [i.e. in the patient's home] that's ... not easy to deal with and you find it stressful and you don't really know what to do. I think it's really important to debrief [smiles] and ... who you do that with is ... I think pretty critical. ... The one ... person I looked after I didn't have

the opportunity to talk to anyone about, and there were some problems in there [i.e. the case]. ... I had some problems with it ... and ... I found that I wrote letters to people about it [smiles] and that was my means of ... sort of de-stressing myself. ... It's unusual. ... I wrote to a friend and I wrote to ... someone I used to work with. ... Two ... letters that I [would] normally have not [written] ... The only reason I wrote was ... because I was feeling ... this stress or this anxiety or this ... I guess bottled up feeling, ... It wasn't the sort of thing that I could have shared with ... either my partner or ... someone that I work with here ... because ... I don't think that they would have understood ... why this situation was stressful. ...

[Carol, GP, age mid-30s; Anglo-Celtic]

The difficulty in conveying meaning was compounded multiple times by the continued relay of information *back and forth* between doctor, patient, family, and other health providers (see also the 'Dynamics of disclosure' section in Chapter 2).

Ambiguity in the location of responsibility

Responsibility for cancer illness and its treatment theoretically lay with either the patient, family, specialist, GP, other allied health personnel, or a combination of these persons. Consensus on how responsibility should be shared, however, was not always ideal, causing considerable uncertainty. From the medical perspective, responsibility had to be defined and negotiated on two levels: that which defined the doctor's role in the multidisciplinary health-care team and which distinguished their own particular responsibilities; and how responsibility was to be shared between the doctor and the particular patient and family.

The multidisciplinary setting has already been shown to be a potential source of conflict between health professionals if management approaches differed within it, or if hierarchical pressure stifled the autonomy of less powerful members of the health team, such as the GP (see Chapter 2 and also: Bosk, 1979 on hierarchy within surgical units; Katz, 1985 on surgeons' perceived vulnerability at losing cancer patients to medical oncologists; and Delvecchio-Good, 1985 on the interaction between experienced, 'old-fashioned' GPs and young, 'high-tech' consultants). Strong (1984) provides a general discussion on the diversity and ambiguity of interdisciplinary relationships that underpin such observations.

Shifting away from interaction across disciplines, the *individual* level of interaction between health-care provider and patient/family also harbours potential ambiguity in terms of the location of responsibility. For instance, 'when the physician assigns a medical diagnosis to a condition that is primarily social, the doctor–patient relationship becomes fraught with ambiguity. The physician ... faces a dilemma: how much of the emotional suffering is his [sic] responsibility to ameliorate? The limits of medical responsibility are poorly defined under such circumstances' (Becker & Nachtigall, 1991: 882). Calnan (1984) echoes similar thoughts. Although cancer is far from a purely 'social' diagnosis, its social, psychological and spiritual impacts are significant, making it highly subject to this form of uncertainty.

As hopes for cure or remission successively waned, specialists progressively (and appropriately) phased themselves out of the process of care, leaving the GPs more and more autonomous in their responsibility. However, while GP care was generally appreciated, sometimes patients and families yearned for specialised, presumably 'better', medical input. It was thus noteworthy that Maria *[Maria, age 69 with breast cancer; Peter, age 74—husband; Greek]*, although she was no longer seeing her consultant, was satisfied that the attending GP was sending her 'papers' (that is, records) to the specialist. This issue, coupled with patient and family anxiety, sometimes lead to role-forcing (Glaser & Strauss, 1965), where the GP was directed to act in ways the patient or family thought appropriate.

Cancer's ambiguities in terms of the end-points and aims of treatment (Freeman, Altice, Betton, Lincoln, & Robbins, 1976) could also create tension and extend role-forcing to the medical profession as a whole, rather than to the individual GP. Carol *[Carol, GP, age mid-30s; Anglo-Celtic]* vividly illustrated this:

CAROL ... he was in his fifties and ... he had a lung cancer but he had been diagnosed about five years before and ... he had spent quite a bit of that time in the United States ... and, clearly in the United States they were very aggressive in terms of ... treatment. And ... this was an extremely difficult relationship because the man ... wanted to be ... actively and aggressively treated. ... The ... thoracic surgeon and chest physicians looking after him ... were saying, ... "Look, you've had everything that you can have" ... and ... he didn't accept it, and his family didn't accept what was going on. ...   *[Carol, GP, age mid-30s; Anglo-Celtic]*

In general, GPs demonstrated a high sense of responsibility for their patients, encapsulated by Theodore's *[Theodore, GP, age 63; Greek]* categorical statement that the GP was the *only* possible case manager in home-based palliative care. However, the sense of responsibility sometimes took its emotional toll when the GP's commitment to the patient blurred their sense of objectivity:

THEODORE ... this closeness [to the patient and family] is very close and ... you have a bit of a cry for a few seconds and then get back to it. ...

[Theodore, GP, age 63; Greek]

Similar uncertainties were voiced by Anastasia *[Anastasia, GP, age 31; Greek]*, who wondered how she would cope emotionally with the inevitable decline in the near future of some of her very old (but currently well) patients.

Technical uncertainty

Bosk (1979) coined the term 'technical error' with specific reference to surgical process. He defined it as a situation where the medical role is performed conscientiously but 'where the skills fall short of what the task requires' (Bosk, 1979: 37–45). Technical uncertainty therefore pertains to the realm of clinical *experience and dexterity*, rather than to the realm of knowledge (even though knowledge is a key prerequisite for technical dexterity). Medico-legal processes, the changing gender composition of the medical workforce, and the medical hierarchy all contributed to GP 'de-skilling', and hence potentially to technical uncertainty, as Byron reflected:

BYRON ... there's been a drift away from the male doctor ... by the female patient, and that's a bit of a shame I guess. ... All the smears and pill prescriptions are associated with the female doctors now and ... not we guys ... . There's more ... media reporting of ... males not being good with ... female patients and ... more importantly, the availability of females—... why not go to a female? ... The females tell the females this is what they should do, and ... [laughs] ... you're up against it if, if you try [last two words softly spoken]. ... The old ladies [however] ... tend to feel comfortable with somebody of more their sort of age. ... This is ... an area too that ... doesn't have that many babies, and of course ... we're losing those; that's another change that's occurred. We don't deliver them any more. We used to get up in the middle of the night, and ... deliver them at the local hospital. The local hospital's been pulled down and, ... you do shared care, and you never get near a delivery suite any more. ... That has probably separated one from ... the younger [patients] ... the way things were twenty years ago. *[Byron, GP, age 57; Anglo-Celtic]*

The described changes with obstetrics and gynaecology apply to nearly all aspects of clinical medicine, where specialist practice encroaches more increasingly on the 'bread and butter' medical territory of the GP (see also Delvecchio-Good, 1985). The rheumatologist increasingly administers joint injections, the general surgeon increasingly performs minor procedures, the paediatrician increasingly looks after normal babies, the psychiatrist undertakes more counselling, and so on.

The impact of this general phenomenon on GP provision of palliative care, however, was not very marked. GPs seemed comfortable with their level of clinical skill, and the progressive attrition of specialist medical input as the illness advanced enabled them to exercise it.

Implications of process–related uncertainty

The complex and emotion–laden nature of process–related uncertainties made them less amenable to control or reversal than pure knowledge-based uncertainty in the individual doctor. This reality is not totally compatible to the silent implications of the patient-centred model, which over-emphasises the control that a GP has in optimising the relationship if they engage the prescribed strategy of the model (see Introduction). Writings which discuss the physician's right to end the doctor–patient relationship if it violated their 'conscientious sense of professional and personal responsibility' (Siegler, 1981) redress the balance by acknowledging the doctor's limited ability to optimise uncertainty and the relationship itself. The legal relevance of these observations is also clear—health-care system structure and the process of doctor–patient interaction are as important as knowledge-based issues in determining medico-legal liability, but are much less understood and far more under-rated.

Inherent medical uncertainty

Another form of uncertainty in cancer care was *inherent* to the illness situation itself, independent of the knowledge, 'framework of operation', or process-related sources of uncertainty outlined above. It existed in two major forms, uncertainty that was inherent to the nature of the illness and its treatment, and uncertainty connected to existential issues of being and identity. These are discussed below.

Inherent uncertainty in the nature of illness and its treatment

Uncertainty could be *inherent in the clinical situation itself.* To illustrate, consider Carol's *[Carol, GP, age mid-30s; Anglo-Celtic]* comments about a confused patient with lung cancer:

> **CAROL** … we looked after this chap for … quite a while, and … eventually he … became quite psychotic … … and … it may have been drug-related or it may have been … well, *there are lots of reasons that it may have been,* [emphasis added, not actual] … but he became quite psychotic and … he did all sorts of bizarre things …
>
> *[Carol, GP, age mid-30s; Anglo-Celtic]*

Medically speaking, the many possible causes of the psychotic state were *well known.* Of those many possible causes (such as electrolyte imbalance, glucose disturbance, hypoxia, infection, cerebral metastases, metabolic disturbances, drug-related effects, emotional disturbance and many others), each could be *simultaneously* active, and each might *fluctuate* over time. The potential combinations of contributing factors were thus vast and temporally variable. The presence or absence of each individual factor was often impossible to determine medically, leaving aside the more complex issue of its relative contribution to the overall state at that point in time. Not even laboratory tests could solve this problem, often because no specific test was available for the given condition (how, for example, could one be tested for emotional disturbance, or some such other disturbance?). False-positive and false-negative results also made the interpretation of tests difficult, as could their performance at an inappropriate phase of the illness. The practical constraints of cost, time and invasiveness also made 'blanket' testing inappropriate and undesirable. It was only *empirical* treatment and examination in hindsight of its effect that subsequently proved or disproved the working hypothesis or hypotheses.

Patients could not always appreciate such difficulty. Their confidence in medical tests caused confusion when they were not employed, or if they were employed but failed to diagnose the problem, as seen with Maria *[Maria, age 69 with breast cancer; Peter, age 74—husband; Greek].* It then became difficult for the doctor to bridge the distance which that created:

> **ELIZABETH** … This lady came in with pleuritic type chest pain, and I thought, well, this obviously needs investigation, particularly with her history of COAD [i.e. chronic obstructive airways disease], … [and] with her … SCC [i.e. squamous cell

carcinoma] of the ano-rectum ... . So ... I did a chest X-ray which showed an opacity adjacent to the right border of the heart. "Could you please follow up with a CT scan?" [said the report], which I did. The CT scan was inconclusive, "Yes, there's a shadow there, we're not really too sure, please repeat in four weeks, four to six weeks". And the daughter got involved and said, "No, no, you know, I want her sent to a surgeon straight away, this is important enough, I don't want to wait a month." And I said, "Look, but even if I sent her to a thoracic surgeon ... they're still going to maybe wait the recommended time". ...

[Elizabeth, GP, age 32; Croatian]

Treatment itself was also inherently uncertain. What, if any, side effects the patient would develop, what course their illness would take or what specific post-operative complications they would suffer could be anticipated to a degree but remained essentially unknown. Inherent uncertainty therefore tended not to create a dilemma about *what* to do, but rather on what the *best* option was. The choice often depended on the subjective feelings of both the doctor and the patient and family.

Existential uncertainty

Adamson (1997: 134–6), drawing upon various traditions in Western philosophy, defined 'existential uncertainty' as that which refers 'to the individual's awareness that his or her future is open and undetermined'. He goes on to say that 'in the medical encounter, existential uncertainty is that form of uncertainty which is experienced privately by the individual patient upon the realisation that the future life of his or her own mind, body and self is in jeopardy' (Adamson, 1997: 134). This type of uncertainty was relevant to the anticipation of future events: there was a marked difference, for example, in what expected medical decline would *actually be like when it happens*, as opposed to what one imagines it might be like *before* it actually happens (Kellehear, 1990). Existential uncertainty thus related to one's sense of being and self that was reflected against the past and projected into the future, a projection that often extended beyond physical death itself.

Existential uncertainty often extended to those around the patient, including the doctor, as noted by Adamson (1997). The 'preferred identities' and 'identity hierarchies' described in patients with declining health (Charmaz, 1990) therefore also had their *equivalents in the treating doctor*. Existential uncertainty in the doctor, for example, contributed to their difficulties in disclosing bad news, and to the tendency of disclosing what they felt the patient wanted to hear or needed to hear (see Chapter 2 for a thorough discussion of disclosure).

As with other types of inherent uncertainty, the ultimate resolution of existential uncertainty was purely at the mercy of time itself—only time would ultimately reveal the real situation of how closely future events would correlate to the way they had been anticipated.

Implications of inherent medical uncertainty

Inherent medical uncertainty manifested itself widely according to the examples provided. As with other forms of uncertainty, the issue was not *whether* it could be abolished (for that was impossible), but *how* it could be best controlled and lived with.

Uncertainty in the negotiation of different paradigms of illness

The Introduction described how medicine became more patient-centred from the mid-twentieth century. This narrowed, but did not bridge, the conceptual gap between medicine and popular lay theories of health and illness. Therefore, although much medical uncertainty lay *within* the boundaries of the biomedical paradigm itself, considerable uncertainty also existed in how to negotiate differences *between* divergent paradigms of illness.

Most GPs were either neutral or encouraging towards other forms of healing, viewing them as *active* adjuncts to conventional medicine, whether the GP believed in them or not. Mainstream Christian principles of illness and healing, for example, coexisted comfortably with the GPs' biomedical background. The same could not be said for other, alternative paradigms of health and illness, which caused awkwardness if they were seen to hinder the mainstream management or exploit the patient's vulnerability:

> **BEN** [Alternative therapies] ... come in to the picture because of the nature of the illness and because of the seriousness of the prognosis. They can't be ignored. ... [cancer illness] exposes a sort of fringe-dwelling medical paramedic, or whatever you call these people ... that ... are in the cancer industry. ... I find them to be

pretty unpleasant people. ... I think some are better than others but ... to me they convey bullshit. I see it in large letters blasted across the sky. ... Because you don't have the answer doesn't necessarily mean that it is a fair thing to ... give your blessing to people ... who have the capacity to rob [patients] ... blind and ... poison them heartily ... *[Ben, GP, age 49; Jewish]*

Other GPs, such as Margarita *[Margarita, GP, age 33; Greek]*, had a stronger leaning to alternative therapies such as acupuncture, vitamin and other nutritional therapy, meditation and yoga. They were often frustrated that patients, especially Greeks, often had more faith in 'conventional' tablets or injections. For such doctors, conventional medicine itself seemed to be an adjunct to more dominant, non-biomedical conceptions of health and illness.

All of the patients here adhered most strongly to conventional treatment, with relatively little use of alternative medicine. Charles *[Charles, age 72 with prostate cancer; Amanda, age 72—wife; Anglo-Celtic]* used acupuncture for supplemental analgesia and mobility, and Panteleimon *[Panteleimon, age 62 with lung cancer; Mary, age 63—wife; Greek]* used the Greek village remedies of cupping and petrol-rubs to the skin (although these were abandoned as his illness progressed). These patients did not make a clear distinction between medical and non-medical forms of healing. Monica *[Monica, age 48 with breast cancer; Alan, age late 50s—husband; Anglo-Celtic]* was an exception. Trained in mathematics and statistics, she knew that the acupuncture, Chinese herbal medicine, and massage that she used were of questionable efficacy for her condition. They were seen as a supplement to more conventional therapy, with hopes for future controlled trials to more objectively study their value.

Implications of uncertainty in the negotiation of different paradigms of illness

It was knowledge of the biomedical paradigm that made it possible to differentiate between biomedical and non-biomedical forms of healing. The biomedical–non-biomedical distinction was therefore felt most acutely by GPs and by patients and families educated in scientific method. Others less familiar with science did not make such distinctions at all. Therefore, if the GP struggled to personally accept patients' alternative therapies, there was the additional dilemma of how to explain this to patients without disturbing the relationship. The reverse, however, was also true. GPs who accepted Christian religious principles (such as Byron *[Byron, GP, age 57; Anglo-Celtic]*) or alternative therapies (such as Margarita *[Margarita, GP, age 33; Greek]*), faced uncertainties as to if, how, when and to what extent to introduce these into clinical management if the patient's stance on them was unclear.

Discussion about *differences* or *clashes* in paradigms, however, should not distract from a broader type of uncertainty about them, namely, a confusion in how to actually define the medical paradigm and distinguish it from non-medical paradigms. Monica *[Monica, age 48 with breast cancer; Alan, age late 50s—husband; Anglo-Celtic]*, for instance, was in favour of using the randomised controlled trial, a biomedical technique, to measure the efficacy of non-biomedical therapies. The entire movement of 'psychoneuroimmunology' (see Hull, 1994) within medicine also similarly aims to rationalise and test *varying* healing paradigms using *biomedical* reasoning and measures. There seems to be an ontological contradiction in such attempts, unless the paradigms are not fundamentally different or mutually exclusive at all.

Moral and emotional uncertainty

GPs found themselves confronted with many emotional and moral dilemmas in palliative care. These related largely to their sense of professional role and duty, their attitudes about death, dying, quality of life and the aims of palliative care (Dozor & Addison, 1992; Freeman et al., 1976), as well as to their own sense of personal vulnerability to terminal illness. As already discussed, many of the emotional and moral dilemmas actually stemmed from *advances* in medical knowledge and technology.

The strong sense of professional duty and responsibility that was socially linked to the doctor's role offered little scope or justification for them to share their feelings and anxieties with the patient or family. However, the necessity of this in cancer illness was quite strong and doctors grappled for the right solution. Sometimes it forced an emotionless approach in a futile attempt to maintain professional control, with disastrous consequences (recall, for instance, the example of a hospital resident's disclosure of cancer to a patient on the ward—see Chapter 2, p. 49). The opposite scenario, however, such as an open confession or release of emotions could also be hazardous. That was especially so if the patient or family were not coping well, and those situations needed a balanced approach:

ALAN Working in a fairly difficult area, he ... you feel that he [the oncologist] is feeling for you and yet he doesn't get out of control. ... I don't know what happens when he goes home to his wife [laughs] but certainly when he's in his surgery he remains in control, ... which, if we're having trouble coping, that's a bit helpful. ... We don't have to help him cope with his problems too [laughs], there's only one of us that ... is in trouble.

[Monica, age 48 with breast cancer; Alan, age late 50s—husband; Anglo-Celtic]

Attaining the right balance was, however, an often uncertain process, and a process difficult to consciously control because of the emotive nature of the situation. Elizabeth *[Elizabeth, GP, age 32; Croatian]* for example, described a consultation where she diagnosed a brain tumour in the daughter of a close friend, and could not hold back the tears, despite her best efforts to do so.

Emotional and moral uncertainties also applied to treatment, where the distinction between usefully prolonging life and unnecessarily prolonging death was blurred (see also Groopman, 1987):

ANASTASIA ... I would say it was ... three to four weeks where I was visiting her daily ... including ... home phone numbers and back up on the weekend if need be. ... So as I said she was an amazingly strong woman. ... And things we'd do like put her on dexamethasone and her jaundice improved. And I was thinking ... , "What are we doing here?" ... *[Anastasia, GP, age 31; Greek]*

Another GP highlighted this dilemma by initially proclaiming that there was 'no such thing as death' (that is, there was no such thing as end-stage illness) but immediately following with a contradictory comment:

THEODORE I've been around a long time, there's no such thing as death. ... I'm sorry I don't ... until I see they've gone yellow, not eating, and then intense pain, [only then] I think ... , "Why the hell have they been kept alive?".

[Theodore, GP, age 63; Greek]

Patients themselves sometimes engaged this debate. For instance, Jane *[Jane, English, age 61 with mycosis fungoides; John, German, age 70—husband]* spoke with favourable allusions to euthanasia (no such allusions were seen in Greek informants, likely due to the Orthodox Christian prohibition of it):

JANE ... I have no intention, especially at sixty-one years of age, to ever suffer like that again [referring to ultraviolet treatment to her skin which had intense side effects]. And if this does deteriorate and take over, I do hope by then Australia has a panel of reliable, sensible humanitarian doctors that would help me to put an end to the suffering. ... Because I have no intentions of suffering right to the end. [pause] One way or another.

[Jane, English, age 61 with mycosis fungoides; John, German, age 70—husband]

As Chapter 2 has shown, GPs were flexible in approaching these and other moral dilemmas, but usually had personal boundaries beyond which no compromise was possible. Unacceptable tasks demanded of them included lying to patients to conceal the diagnosis; accepting extra money offered by Greek patients to buy 'better' care (as commonly occurred in Greece); organising inappropriate investigations because of patient and family pressure; and requests for euthanasia. Such moral stances often threatened the stability of the GP's relationship with the patient and family. Siegler (1981) again reminds one that, ultimately, a realistic option left to the doctor in cases of non-compromise is to hand the case over to someone else.

Implications of moral and emotional uncertainty

Bosk (1979), in his study of the function of surgical units in a major United States tertiary hospital, distinguished moral dilemmas on two major planes. There were those pertaining to the clinical situation itself (such as the question of how aggressively to treat severely malformed neonates who had little chance of long-term survival), and those pertaining to the individual doctor (Bosk, 1979). The latter were concerned with the sincerity and the application with which the doctor executed their duties; in other words, they reflected the doctor's sense of commitment to the patient. Surgical superiors were intolerant of poor commitment to patients but were understanding of inherent moral issues in practice that complicated decision making and caused emotional stress (Bosk, 1979).

The relevant point here is that similar observations were made on how families reacted to the moral and emotional uncertainties of GPs. Such uncertainties were more likely to be accepted if families felt that their doctor was genuinely committed to them, even though their viewpoints on a particular issue might have differed.

Uncertainty in the clinical context: an overview

Having described and discussed the major categories of medical uncertainty as summarised in Box 3.1, a step back is taken to overview the entire place of uncertainty in the clinical process. Subsequently, its overall implications for medical power and the doctor–patient relationship will be discussed.

Effects of medical uncertainty on professional role and identity

A lone discussion of medical uncertainty underemphasises the place of medical *certainty* in the clinical process. Authors such as Atkinson (1984), Calnan (1984) and, to a smaller degree, Light (1979) have all noted the artificiality of viewing medical uncertainty in isolation from medical *certainty*. It is the nature of certainty that defines uncertainty, and therefore 'issues of "certainty" and "uncertainty" are not mutually exclusive' but are instead 'two modes or attitudes towards knowledge and action' (Atkinson, 1984: 954). Fox's (1957) emphasis on knowledge-based uncertainty has been criticised by Atkinson (1984: 954) for viewing the medical practitioner as a scientist who is 'striving to "falsify" and test their hypotheses to the limit', rather than the pragmatist that they really are, 'content to work within the conceptual bounds of (their) given paradigm'.

In the pragmatic nature of the clinical encounter, the nature of medical certainty not only defines and characterises the different types of uncertainty, but also forms the framework in which such uncertainties are tackled. Clinical routines, for instance, inject structure and order even to situations that are uncertain (Adamson, 1997; Calnan, 1984). Bosk (1979) observed different routines in surgical practice between differing consultant surgeons for the same condition (such as different investigative methods, different methods of wound closure, and others). It was the respective routine itself that generated certainty. Differences in approach did not produce anxiety over which one of them was best (which was unknown in the empirical sense), because each approach seemed to produce adequate results. The key issue in uncertainty that led to adverse results then became one of 'distinguishing between what was a reasonable treatment option that subsequent events proved wrong, and a course of action that was indefensible given the facts at hand, an *error*' (Bosk, 1979:

24). Even an error, however, could at least be *morally* defensible if it was made in honest good faith and in a genuine effort to help the patient (Bosk, 1979).

The complex nature of the clinical encounter meant that *both* practical and theoretical reasoning held important and necessary places within it (Atkinson, 1984). This solidifies and supports Calnan's (1984) conclusion that clinical uncertainty does not often present a major threat to professional identity and autonomy. The reason for this is that uncertainty is not generally subject to statistical scrutiny and therefore is not always framed as having a precise, or mathematically-derived, solution. Rather, medical uncertainty is expected, and there are, in many instances, routines for *dealing* with it (though not necessarily *solving* it).

Bosk (1979) went further in his observations by noting that both the trainee and the consultant surgeons' confession of clinical uncertainty and difficulty to their colleagues served to *strengthen* their fellowship with them. That was because all could identify with such problems. The GP's need to 'debrief' with professional colleagues was a parallel in this study. The relevant point here is that not only was uncertainty *not* medically demoralising, but it also contributed towards *defining* the doctor's sense of professional role and duty.

So much for the effects of medical uncertainty upon professional identity and authority. However, how did this translate to the interaction between doctor, patient and family?

The relativity and paradox of uncertainty in clinical interaction

Chapter 2 concluded with the suggestion that medical uncertainty could be a major impediment to doctor–patient compatibility and therefore to the therapeutic relationship as a whole. The different types of medical uncertainty that have been described, the intricate manner in which they related to each other, and their potential to fluctuate and coexist in many different combinations lends considerable support to such a conclusion. However, the link between uncertainty and compatibility was *not unidirectional*. That is, uncertainty did not influence compatibility in an independent manner, but, rather, was itself *affected by it*. For example, a compatible relationship between doctor and patient might ease the tension about uncertainty because of an enhanced mutual understanding between them regarding each other's predicament. Conversely, such a relationship might also make uncertainty harder to bear by both because of the heightened sense of loss that it could engender in each of them.

It was such a dynamic and variable relationship between medical uncertainty and doctor–patient compatibility that explained why the *universal* presence of uncertainty did not uniformly destroy trust and closeness in the doctor–patient relationship. Rather, it could diversely effect the medical power that emanated from an individual doctor. Such effects on medical power were not simply related to the ability of doctors to either *avoid* or *control* uncertainty (both options were often impossible), as the doctor's status could remain intact or even become *enhanced* in the presence of unavoidable or uncontrollable uncertainty. Conversely, there were instances where medical power was destroyed if uncertainty could not be avoided or controlled.

Examples where medical power remained intact and was even enhanced despite uncertainty were numerous, and manifested in different ways. Patient and family confidence could be enhanced in the knowledge that their doctor was actively interested in their condition, as seen in the relationship between Jane *[Jane, English, age 61 with mycosis fungoides; John, German, age 70—husband]* and her dermatologist. Clare *[Clare, age 65 with stomach cancer; Michael, age 67—husband; Anglo-Celtic]* and Charles *[Charles, age 72 with prostate cancer; Amanda, age 72—wife; Anglo-Celtic]* appreciated the caring administered by their respective GPs, despite the terminal nature of their illness. Barbara and her husband Dimitri *[Barbara, age 48 with cervical cancer; Dimitri, age 53—husband; Greek]*, who benefited greatly from palliative surgery to relieve tumour-induced urinary obstruction, were greatly impressed at what medicine was able to achieve in an illness situation that could only be negative. Such positive feelings in patient and family empowered doctors and their own sense of control over the illness. In fact, somewhat paradoxically, the more the GP immersed themselves into the insurmountable uncertainty and emotional challenges present in palliative care (rather than resisting them), the more satisfaction and motivation they received:

> **ANDREW** ... I think it's the motivation that you're caring and concerned for the, for your patients, for the person that's going through this particular suffering and ... , who really is as I see it probably feeling very, very alone in the world and very, very frightened ... and I think ... I don't think there could be anything more frightening than that, ... than to feel alone. ... Even when you are surrounded by your family and whatever, but also people do abandon you at this time. So I guess I feel very committed to people like this because they're going through a very difficult predicament. *[Andrew, GP, age early 40s; Greek]*

Examples where medical power was completely dismantled because uncertainty could not be overcome or appropriately managed were also numerous. The disintegration of the relationship between Maria *[Maria, age 69 with breast cancer; Peter, age 74—husband; Greek]* and the original Greek GP who failed to diagnose her breast cancer was one example. Other examples of relationships that were terminated included that between Paraskevi *[Paraskevi, age 48 with cervical cancer; Mark, age 23—son; Greek]* and the hospital that initially assessed her for cervical cancer (Chapter 2, p. 92), and also that between Monica *[Monica, age 48 with breast cancer; Alan, age late 50s—husband; Anglo-Celtic]* and the general surgeon, whose approach seemed excessively and haphazardly interventionist to her (Chapter 2, p. 79).

The notion of *advantageous* elements in uncertainty was found to be an important factor that could reduce its threat. The section on 'Cancer as gain' in Chapter 1 described how positive factors could spring from cancer, especially renewed closeness between family members. Many of the GPs also used uncertainty to positive advantage in a realistic manner according to the particular circumstances. Chapter 2 gave several examples of this. Uncertainty of negative progress, for instance, could at times be realistically emphasised more strongly than uncertainty about positive progress. At other times, uncertainty could be placed in the hands of the Almighty, stripping it of its threat and sanctifying it instead, rendering it safe and acceptable. Additionally, the view of uncertainty as an inevitable part of life also rendered it natural and expected, thereby transforming it into certainty.

In summary, then, uncertainty itself, like medical power, was a relative and sometimes paradoxical phenomenon. The social interaction between doctor and patient ultimately determined the framework within which uncertainty and compatibility were defined and identified. Therefore, uncertainty in itself was not seen to be as strong a *determinant* of doctor–patient compatibility as the conclusion to Chapter 2 hypothesised, but rather a *reflection* of it. The issue that remains is how to link the analysis of the two. The notion of 'distance' between doctor and patient provides a potential avenue towards this aim.

Conclusion: the concept of doctor–patient distance

The notion of a 'distance' between doctor and patient was strongly pervasive in the interview data. This did not only reflect the obvious difference in social status and vulnerability that distinguished the doctor's predicament from that of the patient. It also incorporated many more subtle parameters at the personal and emotional level, and even issues such as the physical distance and spacing between doctor and patient when they were together. In striving to be compatible, participants in the relationship had to simultaneously preserve their own social roles and identities against the effects of medical uncertainty and other threats. Such a quest to preserve roles and identities limited the closeness that could be attained in a therapeutic relationship. Uncertainty about what an 'appropriate distance' was or meant also affected the compatibility that could be achieved.

The concept of distance was therefore important because it *simultaneously united issues of uncertainty with issues of compatibility* into the core task that was unconsciously undertaken by everyone involved in the therapeutic relationship alike (doctor, patient, carer, allied health professional, and other personnel). The core task was that of attaining an *'optimal distance'* in their relationships with each other. The notion is dynamic, emphasising evolution in the doctor–patient relationship over time, and is therefore compatible with the view of the clinical process as an 'unfolding event', where earlier events determine the nature of subsequent ones (Fisher, 1984).

By unifying the issues of compatibility and uncertainty over the sequential passage of time, the notion of 'distance' could shed light upon several key questions, such as: How, when and to what degree could a stable doctor–patient relationship tolerate medical uncertainty? Could a particular doctor–patient relationship tolerate certain kinds of medical uncertainty above others? How easily could uncertainty-related damage to a therapeutic relationship be reversed? Such questions probe at the core issues of medical power.

The next chapter will further expound and examine the issue of distance in the doctor–patient relationship. After this, an overall response to the problems posed about medical power in the Introduction can be provided.

4

Distance, ownership and role reversal in clinical relationships

Chapter 3 concluded that medical uncertainty was often a *reflection* of doctor–patient compatibility and harmony rather than a *determinant* of it. Further, the notion of 'distance' between doctor and patient formed a means of linking the issues of compatibility and uncertainty over the sequential passage of time.

This chapter re-examines the interaction between medical and non-medical worlds with specific reference to 'distance' between individuals. It attempts to consolidate and unite the diverse issues that generate interpersonal distance (as seen in Chapter 2), themselves tormented by clinical uncertainty (seen in Chapter 3), to the paradoxical ability of doctor and patient to bond despite such difficulties. It begins with a brief review of the notion of distance itself, and refines this discussion by introducing the reciprocal notion of ownership. It specifically examines the difficulty in minimising distance but simultaneously avoiding excessive ownership in the quest to optimise doctor–patient compatibility. The chapter then discusses properties of ownership and distance when the direction of care is reversed—that is, when patient and family offer care to the doctor. The implications of these findings for an understanding of compatibility between doctor and patient, for the distinctiveness of their roles and, more broadly, for medical power itself are discussed in conclusion.

Interpersonal distance between doctor and patient

The distance between doctor and patient (or between any persons involved in the illness) is a concept denoting the degree of *separation* that existed between them. Distance could potentially be constructed and analysed around a countless number of different and individual parameters. These include roles (that is, doctor versus patient), knowledge, socio-economic status, age, gender, culture, religion, actual physical distance and positioning between doctor and patient during their encounters, and so on.

Many of these parameters, as seen in Chapter 3, were completely *external* to the doctor–patient relationship, often influencing it as strongly as did personal interaction within the relationship. For example, gender, language and culture, or health-system structure presented issues of distance in their own right, being primarily unrelated to any interaction between doctor and patient (although such interaction could subsequently modify or refine them). They instead reflected broad, social ideas of appropriateness within the doctor–patient relationship.

The key aim of all participants in the illness was to *minimise* or *optimise* the distance between themselves and others in order to facilitate the process of care. Distance was thus a dynamic concept, temporally variable according to how it was modified by interaction. Despite the presence of many types of distance, three main categories of distance seemed most crucial to the nature, function, and distribution of power within the doctor–patient relationship. These were professional distance, social distance and emotional distance. They encompassed many of the individual areas of distance already mentioned (for example, social distance incorporated gender, cultural, religious and socio-economic distance). It is to these three key categories of distance that specific attention is now turned. Their separate discussion should not suggest a mutual exclusiveness; rather, they influenced and affected each other.

Professional distance

Professional distance refers to the gap in authority, role, knowledge and expertise between the doctor and patient in relation to illness. 'The doctor as a man [sic] apart from those he treats has been a recurrent theme ...' in medical and sociological literature (Stimson & Webb, 1975: 59). The use of the title 'Doctor' by both doctors and patients illustrated such distance, as did the word 'patient' (alternative words such as 'client' or 'consumer' were not used by any of the GPs and only rarely by patients and carers in this study). Common GP language such as '*I sent her off ...*', '*I did* a ...', '*They needed* a ...' also emphasised distance in terms of roles and responsibilities. The outward expression of this distance could be grounded on pure medical science, and therefore be impersonal, or it could be patient-centred and more personalised.

It was precisely such distance in terms of medical knowledge and expertise that formed the basis of the doctor–patient relationship. As such, this distance was often actively welcomed. People *wanted* their doctors to be highly skilled and caring, and were prepared to tolerate considerable inconveniences as a result:

> **ALAN** He is a caring GP ... he is not a machine GP—you don't get your five minutes and out the door, five minutes out the door, five minutes out the door. He has a booking system that can get to be an hour and a half or two hours out of kilter by about two o'clock in the afternoon ... and by the evening ... it's just almost impossible to know whether he'll be catching up or falling behind or where he'll be. And, when you're as sick as Monica you can't ... be seen [last words unclear] in this manner. ... On the other hand, from a customer's point of view, you notice we haven't changed away from him ... because if a patient needs not the five minutes but three quarters of an hour, he gets three quarters of an hour ... and he will be looked after ... so ... , you know, ... you put up with the messes ... as well as the good bits.
>
> *[Monica, age 48 with breast cancer; Alan, age late 50s—husband; Anglo-Celtic]*

Such professional distance was variable in both its inward and outward manifestations. The inward manifestation was affected, for example, by whether the doctor was the patient's '*main GP*' *[Frank, GP, age early 30s; Anglo-Celtic]* as opposed to the temporary GP. Although the temporary GP could be fully patient-centred and committed to the patient, they did not fully 'own' them, nor did they wish to—the patient 'belonged' to another GP. This relationship therefore differed in essence from that between the patient and their regular GP. Temporary patients were called 'the' patient, rather than 'my' patient, and likewise temporary GPs were called 'the' doctor, rather than 'my' doctor (see Chapter 1 on the 'partnership emphasis' in management).

The outward manifestation of professional distance was also variable. The older Anglo-Celtic informants, for example, grew up knowing doctors to be authoritative, respected and predominantly male. Although they appreciated modern, more open medical relationships, the narrowing of professional distance generated by the patient–centred clinical model was often simultaneously uncomfortable:

> **MICHAEL** ... ... doctors have always been someone to be respected. And I've always called a doctor a doctor, see? Now, Dr Jones likes to be called Karen, ... you see. Do you think I can call her ... Dr Karen? I cannot. [both laugh]. I cannot for the life of me, and every time we go out I say, "Thank you Dr Jones". "Karen", [she says], you know. [both laugh] ... I just can't ... I'll get it down to Dr Karen but I just can't say ... [Karen] ... , you know, like without being a doc [myself] see, because I had trouble with my leg when I was a little fella, you know, and, ... [our] family doctor [was] ... *Doctor* Jakeson [emphasised] ...
> *[Clare, age 65 with stomach cancer; Michael, age 67—husband; Anglo-Celtic]*

These informants were most comfortable with a distinct professional formality and authority in the doctor's role; challenging medical authority, role-forcing and medical litigation were therefore foreign concepts. Michael and Clare *[Clare, age 65 with stomach cancer; Michael, age 67—husband; Anglo-Celtic]* did not understand their surgeon's explanation of a planned laparotomy ('... *of course it was all over mum's head and everything, you know* ...'), but did not even ask him for clarification.

GPs themselves generally favoured the patient–centred approach as a means of narrowing professional distance, although it sometimes generated too uncomfortable a familiarity. The doctor sometimes had to safeguard professional distance by dressing more formally, by placing *physical* distance between themselves and the patient (as did Byron *[Byron, GP, age 57; Anglo-Celtic]* and Andrew *[Andrew, GP, age early 40s; Greek]* in sitting on the opposite side of the consulting desk), or by using their title more formally:

> **ELIZABETH** ... With younger Anglo-Saxon patients ... well I'm just ... the same person as them [i.e. young], ... but they don't hold doctors with the same esteem or respect, I believe, as maybe what they [i.e. society in general] did once. And [I find the same] talking to the other doctors here ... who are much older than myself, they're fifty plus. ... And also, personally, I object to the fact that they [i.e. patients] use my first name, they call me by my first name. I personally don't like that, because I don't introduce myself using my first name.
> *[Elizabeth, GP, age 32; Croatian]*

The issue of professional distance was also made more delicate and complex by the existence of a medical hierarchy. Patients, particularly

Greek patients, often saw specialist approaches as more active than GP treatment. Andrew's *[Andrew, GP, age early 40s; Greek]* reflections of his Greek patients were particularly revealing:

> **ANDREW** ... the GP is seen as not being an expert and therefore not as good as a specialist. I do feel that very much, very often. ... I suppose [it's] more so with particular patients; not everybody is like that ... I had a guy yesterday who came in for some blood tests for his cholesterol ... and he said, "... I've had some problems ... send me to a urologist, I need to have my prostate tested". I said, "But I can do that for you". ... And his wife jumped in and said, "Oh no, no ... I think its probably best to go to a specialist. Don't you think so?" I said, "Well, okay, ... if that's what you want, that's fine". But I said, "In any case, since we are doing blood tests, I'll do the blood test for the prostate ... and the specialist can examine it", ... and they were happy with that ... So yeah, ... people certainly do not have a concept of what a GP does ... what his scope is. ... Patients don't often ask, "Can you do this, doctor?", but they'll say, "I need to see such and such a specialist". ... Certainly there is an attitude that GPs are second rate, in inverted commas. *[Andrew, GP, age early 40s; Greek]*

Such difficulty might have reflected the absence of a GP-equivalent in Greece itself. Anastasia's *[Anastasia, GP, age 31; Greek]* medical cousin in Greece, a vascular surgical trainee, could not understand the notion of a GP, because '*you've just got to specialise*':

> **ANASTASIA** ... I remember when I visited Greece a couple of years back [he'd] ... say, "Well, what have you just done?", and I'd just done a cas [i.e. casualty or emergency medicine] term and he goes, "Well ... what does this mean? ... What's a cas term?", and I'd say [what it was] ... So he basically gave me a scenario [of what I'd do] if some guy came in with a DVT [i.e. a deep venous thrombosis] and it was in the middle of the night. And I said, "Well, if it was in the middle of the night ... you'd assume that's what it is and ... you'd start heparinising ...", and then he goes, "You do?! You'd do that?!!" [both laugh loudly] He goes, "My gosh, oh, you're good!!", you know ... [interviewer and Anastasia still laughing]. But there [in Greece] ... even [with] the concept of ... cas[ualty] ... the doctors there do some sort of triage ... and then they call the big guys in. *[Anastasia, GP, age 31; Greek]*

Such lack of trust and confidence in the GP often saw Greek patients go from '*doctor to doctor and from alternative medicine to alternative medicine*', as Theodore *[Theodore, GP, age 63; Greek]* put it. The patient-centred approach theoretically facilitated this behaviour by sanctioning the patient's freedom to tailor their management accordingly. (The Medicare system and the oversupply of GPs in metropolitan regions likewise allowed this to occur.) This frustrated GPs:

> **ANASTASIA** ... They're [i.e. older Greeks] not very good at seeing their GP as their advocate, of someone who can look after them in the big hospital. And I think ... it's hard to impress that on them. ... Whereas I think non-Greek speaking patients find that a lot easier. A much easier concept to have, ... 'cause they'd rather be out of the big hospitals, ... they'd rather be looked after by their GP and rather be at home and stuff, you know.   *[Anastasia, GP, age 31; Greek]*

Despite their tendency to undervalue the GP role, however, Greeks often valued *individual* GPs for particular skills, especially those relating to early diagnosis, efficient treatment, and apparent concern for the patient. Even then, however, they could remain selective in what they presented with:

> **THEODORE** ... They might come to me ... for gynaecology ... and go to Vafiadis for ... arthritis. ... And they wouldn't tell you that. But you accept that. They just know something about it because ... [I've] treated somebody for [a] gynaecological condition, Vafiadis for a broken leg, and he's an expert on this area and (I'm an expert on mine), [and] that sort of goes on.
> **INTERVIEWER** Word gets around, do you think?
> **THEODORE** Oh, absolutely. What happens in Frankston, you'll hear in Coburg by the next day. Absolutely. ... If someone's got a headache and they find a cancer of the brain in Frankston, within twenty-four hours you get millions of people running up [to Frankston] with headaches [saying] ... "We heard about this patient [you] were treating."   *[Theodore, GP, age 63; Greek]*

Older Anglo-Celtic informants, in contrast to the Greek-Australians, usually made little distinction between the value of the GP compared to the specialist, and, if they did, it often *favoured* the GP. For example:

> **JANE** ... if I talk ... from a psychological point of view, the skin specialists really don't know what I'm saying. ... But a general practitioner has a larger spectrum, ... and is able to ... put them into categories, and say, "Well, really I think you ought to go to this specialist or that specialist", but I can't see a specialist being able to do that. ... The general practitioner is ... able to cope, to categorise ... much better. ... And they're ... more interested in the *family* [emphasised] background too ... they bring that into it as well. ... I've got the feeling it's "Treat the patient and not the disease", ... more with the general practitioner.
> *[Jane, English, age 61 with mycosis fungoides; John, German, age 70—husband]*

Finally, the influence of a medical hierarchy was not only located in the social consciousness of patients and their families, but also operated within the medical profession itself, making GPs on occasions tend to feel inferior to their specialist colleagues (see Chapter 3, p. 107).

Social distance

Social distance incorporated those factors that shaped interpersonal interaction in more routine or 'everyday' contexts, as opposed to the highly specific context of the clinical consultation. Although such factors are examined from within the professional context of the doctor–patient relationship, they were not specific to it.

The very location and organisation of the general practice sent out silent social messages that influenced the type of clientele attending the clinic (Stimson & Webb, 1975). Issues such as practice aesthetics, billing procedures, the socio-economic status of the practice's suburb, its hours of opening and the type of services provided were all important in this respect, as was medical insurance. Private health insurance allowed the patient to select their specialist doctor(s) and also short-circuited lengthy appointment and treatment delays inherent in the public health system, thereby facilitating a greater sense of control. Only two participating families, *[Monica, age 48 with breast cancer; Alan, age late 50s—husband; Anglo-Celtic]* and *[Barbara, age 48 with cervical cancer; Dimitri, age 53— husband; Greek]*, had private health insurance.

Gender-related issues were also an important component of social distance. Byron *[Byron, GP, age 57; Anglo-Celtic]* noted that most young females attended female doctors, especially for obstetric and gynaecological problems. This could possibly be linked to an increasingly greater availability of female doctors or the politicising of women's health by the feminist movement. However, it may have reflected genuine differences in the way male and female doctors practised clinical medicine. Research evidence on the latter point is conflicting (West, 1993). There were no impressions here of gender-specific distinctions in the way the GP informants practised palliative care.

Older Anglo-Celtic female patients, being accustomed to male GPs in their youth, did not show a distinct preference for female GPs, as noted by Byron *[Byron, GP, age 57; Anglo-Celtic]*, whose male *and* female patient population was ageing along with himself. Gender issues among Greek patients, however, seemed a more potent determinant of distance. Many of Margarita's *[Margarita, GP, age 33; Greek]* Greek patients only attended her for Papanicolaou smear tests, having another doctor, often a male, for their more general health care. Gender bias by male patients also made female GPs potentially more vulnerable to intimidation or disrespect. Anastasia [*Anastasia, GP, age 31; Greek*] felt this among many older Greek men:

> **ANASTASIA** ... it was interesting ... working ... for Alexi [a solo male Greek GP] ... that sometimes you would get the very arrogant men who [laughs] ... [thought], you know, "Oh, a female GP, oh yeah, you've got Buckleys'", you know, "I'm really going to take you seriously", sort of thing. You know, very, very arrogant men; but that doesn't happen very often. *[Anastasia, GP, age 31; Greek]*

Gender distance was also an issue *within* Greek households. The Southport Hospice, for example, noted that they almost never bathed Greek males under their care because their wives usually did this. However, they routinely bathed Greek females because their husbands were uncomfortable or unwilling to do so.

Optimising gender distance was therefore complex but perceived medical skill, trust, and familiarity with the patient seemed important factors in this task. Irrespective of these, however, precautionary actions are now increasingly appearing in standard practice, such as the use of female chaperones by male doctors in gynaecological or obstetric examinations.

With such a strong cultural component inherent in the notion of power and gender, the question also arose of the importance of cultural compatibility *per se* between doctor and patient for the stability of their relationship. An Australian national multicultural health conference concluded that cultural compatibility could *not* be replaced by cross-cultural awareness alone:

> *The focus on culture in relation to equity in service provision is accompanied by the pursuit of 'cultural awareness' and the development of 'culturally aware' health professionals. This is a rather paternalistic model, which posits knowledge of culture of the 'clients' within the relatively powerful service providers. It is most likely invalid for a number of reasons, not the least of which is the fact that the majority of health practitioners are unlikely to be more than dimly aware of their own culture let alone the hundreds of cultures and sub-cultures potentially presenting through their clients.*
>
> (Southern Sydney Area Health Service, 1994: 18)

A proposed solution to this pseudo-dilemma was to provide culturally appropriate care to people from non-English-speaking backgrounds by increasing recruitment of overseas-trained doctors to Australia (Southern Sydney Area Health Service, 1994). Such an assessment discounted personal dimensions in interaction, devalued the idea of multiculturalism, did not consider potential cross-cultural clashes between such medical recruits and the wider multicultural community, and was not supported by the informant data.

In this study, many Anglo-Celtic informants had close relationships with GPs from non-English-speaking backgrounds. Additionally, most Greek informants did not have GPs with a Greek background, often using children or other relatives as interpreters if needed. Such established doctor–patient relationships were valued and worked well. Two Greek families, *[Maria, age 69 with breast cancer; Peter, age 74—husband; Greek]* and *[Panteleimon, age 62 with lung cancer; Mary, age 63—wife; Greek]* specifically left their Greek-background GPs for non-Greek GPs. For Katerina *[George, age mid-50s with lung cancer; Katerina, age —wife; Greek]* whose mother had recently died in appalling conditions in an Athens hospital, the presence of *any doctor at all* was considered a blessing.

The data suggested that bridging cultural and ethnic distance seemed to depend most heavily on the ability to communicate in the same *language*. As seen elsewhere (Naish, Brown & Denton, 1994), it was language, lying behind a cultural guise, that was the key issue in such settings. Likewise, differences in religious affiliation *per se* did not generate much distance between doctor and patient. Occasional exceptions were seen, as with Barbara and Dimitri's *[Barbara, age 48 with cervical cancer; Dimitri, age 53—husband; Greek]* refusal of needed blood transfusions, as they were both Jehovah's Witnesses. Signed statements releasing medical staff of responsibility were sufficient to contain medical dissent, although they did not eliminate it. More generally, however, religion was used by some GPs to infuse meaning into negative or uncertain situations, thereby reducing the threat of the illness and helping to optimise distance between themselves and the family.

Narrowing of social distance could also be induced by the home-based setting of the consultations. There, the doctor was more exposed to the hospitality of the family, evidenced through their offerings of tea and sweets (as described by Andrew *[Andrew, GP, age early 40s; Greek]*), garden-grown vegetables (as described by Carol *[Carol, GP, age mid-30s; Anglo-Celtic]*), flowers or other gifts. While often welcomed, such actions could lead to more involved offerings such as casual invitations for coffee or even invitations to important family celebrations like weddings or baptisms (as described by Anastasia *[Anastasia, GP, age 31; Greek]*). The doctor therefore had to be guarded and prepared to limit the degree to which such social distance was narrowed.

Emotional distance

The notion of distance also applied to the more personal and emotional elements of relationships between people. At the root of emotional distance was the fundamental difference in vantage points from which cancer illness was lived: the patient actually *had* it, while the GP merely *treated* it. Chapter 3 showed that emotional feelings were located beyond the scope of linguistic expression, therefore making it difficult to bridge emotional distance.

GPs expended considerable energy in understanding and pleasing the patient, consistent with the dictates of the patient-centred approach—dictates also inherent in cultural awareness models (see the Introduction) and models of dying (see Kellehear, 1990). These, however, could create confusion, conflict and moral dilemmas in care without being equipped to solve them (recall the issues involved in disclosure from Chapter 2). Involving the patient in clinical decision making might be seen as a sign of medical uncertainty or that there was little more useful intervention available, as seen with Maria *[Maria, age 69 with breast cancer; Peter, age 74—husband; Greek]*. Patient centredness also often brought GPs personally closer to the sense of their own mortality, causing discomfort and much contemplation and personal reflection. It also created moral dilemmas in practical terms, as seen with Carol *[Carol, GP, age mid-30s; Anglo-Celtic]*, who had to take her infant son with her to an after hours home call because no one was available to baby sit.

The patient-centred approach also tested the degree to which GPs were prepared to compromise their own outlooks on the clinical situation. Critical differences between GP and patient views were often difficult to resolve. GPs would not travel beyond personal boundaries to satisfy patient or family desires, such as lying about the diagnosis, accepting extra money to provide 'better' care, or ordering inappropriate tests. All of these could heighten emotional tension in the relationship.

Additionally, the patient and family were socially sanctioned to openly express emotional sorrow within the clinical relationship (it was not rare, for instance, for patients or family members to cry occasionally). The strong sense of professional duty and responsibility linked to the GP's role, however, hindered an open revelation of their emotions. As discussed in

Chapter 3 (under 'Moral and emotional uncertainty'), that was not always compatible with the stresses of cancer care. Births and deaths were perhaps the only occasions that *called for* and *sanctioned* an open display of emotion between doctor and family:

> **ANASTASIA** ... The only time that patients seem to feel comfortable about kissing you are at births and deaths [laughs], you know what I mean? ... I think that's the only way that they can show it and they sort of ... peck you on the cheek and say, "Wow, thanks for being here", when it's a delivery or ... you know or, ... or they actually feel comfortable giving you sort of physical contact at ... that time I think, and, ... I suppose as a doctor ... too, I mean ... it's a lot easier to hug someone who's partner's just died than ... [at other times] ... [where] ... okay, you might do a supportive touch and counselling and stuff, but ... that comes out more [in these situations]. *[Anastasia, GP, age 31; Greek]*

Emotional distance was also brought about by the difficulty of appreciating the evolution of another's emotions. Even patient-centred doctors struggled to appreciate the active emotional work and preparation of their patients (see also Stimson & Webb, 1975), which differed from appreciating the more mechanical tasks of making an appointment and waiting to see the doctor (see also Strong, 1979 on the latter tasks in paediatric outpatient settings). Simple preparations such as showering and grooming before presenting to the clinic were examples of such emotional preparation. Such preparation also involved very careful planning and rehearsal:

> **FIELD NOTES** I arrived early and sat in the waiting room for half an hour, listening and looking at what people did. Shortly after I arrived, an older man with his adult daughter had come in to see Byron [Dr Barnes] at 2.50 p.m. for a 2.45 p.m. appointment. They waited fifteen minutes before being called. The young lady spoke extensively to her father about his symptoms and wanted to accompany him to see the doctor [who was always referred to as Dr Barnes] so as to explain exactly what had happened to her father. She planned to leave the consulting room when it was time for his examination. She also picked up two prescriptions for her mother, which were waiting for collection at the reception desk. Father and daughter both struggled to decipher the illegible handwriting on them, but failed. They also discussed how many doctors they thought were on duty, and the daughter also spoke about the receptionist who had earlier that day made their appointment. She was no longer on duty, and the father couldn't recall her, so his

daughter described her to him—the one with long, dark hair, the newer one who was tall and who'd come out from England recently. To her frustration, she couldn't remember her name. This showed the special place or prominence that everyone in the clinic had to patients, a fact not often perceived by the staff themselves.

[Byron, GP, age 57; Anglo-Celtic]

The barrier that hindered a fuller appreciation by doctors and practice staff was their *familiarity* with the general practice *routine*. The relative rapidity of ten- to fifteen-minute consultations, time constraints, and the GP's simultaneous involvement in a score of other doctor–patient relationships, each with its own demands, could blur how unique the encounter was to the individual patient. All of these factors explained why routine procedures, such as minor surgery and injections, were often recalled vividly by patients (often many decades after the event), whereas to the GP they were long forgotten because they were routine, performed often on many people, and therefore relatively devoid of distinction.

Refining the concept of distance: the notion of ownership

The discussion of distance thus far has been insufficient to achieve the key aim of linking a positive doctor–patient compatibility to the universal problem of uncertainty. To the contrary, its complexity might suggest that such a link is impossible, given the ubiquitous forms of distance present within the three key categories discussed above. How, after all, could *all* those forms of distance be successfully bridged between individuals who had their own, personal illness vantage point and who defined distance in their own, unique way? Additionally, how did the three main categories of distance (professional, social, and emotional), which were not mutually exclusive, relate to each other in terms of their respective importance and effect upon the 'overall distance' felt between doctor and patient?

Paradoxically, it was this very complexity in the nature of distance that harboured the solution to these problems. The key point was that distance was *not necessarily a negative phenomenon*, and could at times even be *advantageous*. Four closely related points were pivotal towards such an understanding (see Box 4.1) and are further examined below.

BOX 4.1 Key issues linking distance to ownership

The co-existence of ownership within the notion of distance
The ability of ownership to bridge 'non-correlating' forms of distance
The need to maintain some distance in order to facilitate ownership
The tension between minimising distance versus avoiding excessive ownership

The coexistence of ownership within the notion of distance

Each category of distance (professional, social, emotional), and each element of distance within that category was intimately entwined with its own notion of *ownership*, with which it *coexisted*. Ownership denoted the sense of *belonging* or *closeness* that was present between doctor and patient. (Ownership also denoted belonging to the illness itself, its therapeutic regimen, and the degree to which that was accepted.)

It was often the seemingly paradoxical coexistence of ownership with distance that *erased* or *nullified* the negative connotations of the latter. Examples are evident in the preceding discussions on the nature of distance. It was, for example, professional distance (in terms of knowledge and expertise) that in itself also simultaneously fuelled the patient's sense of professional ownership of the doctor, and likewise the doctor's sense of ownership of the patient. Each referred to the other as '*my* doctor', and '*my* patient', respectively, not '*the* doctor' and '*the* patient'. This was consistent with the writing of Silverman (1987) and Maseide (1991), who showed that the distinctiveness of the doctor's role, with its associated power, could strengthen the doctor–patient relationship through the sense of confidence and trust that it engendered. The story of Maria *[Maria, age 69 with breast cancer; Peter, age 74—husband; Greek]*, who had great confidence and respect in the GP who diagnosed her breast cancer, illustrated this point well. The doctor's diagnostic skill, which emphasised knowledge and status (and therefore the professional distance between himself and Maria), *generated* a sense of professional ownership.

Another example was provided by Alan *[Monica, age 48 with breast cancer; Alan, age late 50s—husband; Anglo-Celtic]* concerning the emotional composure and objectivity of Monica's oncologist, which comprised a form of emotional distance. It was precisely the maintenance of such an emotional distance that allowed the family to cope, thereby generating a sense of emotional ownership and attachment for the oncologist (which likely, in turn, also assisted the oncologist's own internal sense of coping).

In a similar fashion, Theodore *[Theodore, GP, age 63; Greek]* cried for his patients *after* they left the consulting room, maintaining an apparent emotional distance so as not to compromise the patient's coping and composure. Distance, therefore, was not as wholly threatening as its superficial appearance might suggest.

The ability of ownership to bridge 'non-correlating' forms of distance

Ownership not only coexisted within its 'correlating' notion of distance (for example, professional ownership within the notion of professional distance, and so on), but could also facilitate ownership across *other* (that is, 'non-correlating') realms of distance. Professional ownership, for example, did not only minimise professional distance but could also nullify or counteract social and emotional distance. This highlighted the dynamic relationship between different forms of distance and also indicated that their effects on the overall sense of doctor–patient belonging were not uniform. Some types of distance were weightier than others according to the unique circumstances of each case.

The example presented above of the closeness of Maria *[Maria, age 69 with breast cancer; Peter, age 74—husband; Greek]* to her diagnosing GP illustrated this point. There, professional ownership (generated *because of* professional distance) was able to facilitate emotional and even social closeness and ownership. When the hope for cure was gone, for instance, and progressive debility forced Maria to seek a GP closer to home, she still wanted to visit the diagnosing GP periodically, just to say *'Hello' [Maria, age 69 with breast cancer; Peter, age 74—husband; Greek]*, and not for any therapeutic reason. It was social and personal contact that she desired.

The relationship between Jane *[Jane, English, age 61 with mycosis fungoides; John, German, age 70—husband]* and her dermatologist also emphasised the dynamic interconnections between 'non-correlating' elements of ownership and distance. The dermatologist, an academic clinician, was mainly interested in Jane's unusual pathology and unexpectedly good response to treatment. Jane herself did not feel that the doctor particularly liked *her*, but his efforts (targeted to her *disease*, not her illness) nevertheless enkindled a confidence within her. This led to a growing sense of emotional ownership between them. (Over time, this would be expected to feed back and modify the doctor's view of the patient, perhaps allowing him to see more of her personal illness rather than her pathological disease.)

The need to maintain some distance in order to facilitate ownership

It was not necessary to completely obliterate distance in order to attain an ideal union or sense of ownership. In the examples above, where ownership was shown to minimise the effects of distance, that ownership itself was founded upon the *presence* of distance. The doctor–patient union *depended* on a certain amount of distance, otherwise its functional character would be lost. Recall the need of the older Anglo-Celtic informants for formality in the interaction, and their inability to use the doctor's first name (p. 128–9). Anastasia's *[Anastasia, GP, age 31; Greek]* experience of having medically treated her mother was another striking example. There, closeness or ownership on the emotional and personal level was so intense that professional ownership, with its implied objectivity, was impossible:

> **ANASTASIA** ... I gave my mum a flu vaccine a couple of years back ... and I reckon I would have given a hundred [flu vaccines] that year and there is a one per cent reaction rate. Well, she got the reaction. ... And it was huge, and ... that was it—I thought, "Well, nothing serious happened", but that was my lesson. I don't even take her blood pressure any more. ... I was really, "Right, I can't treat you. I just don't want the [responsibility] ...", ... And I said to her, "Oh Mum ... does it hurt?" "Oh", she goes, "it doesn't hurt, it doesn't hurt", and you could see ... it was killing her! [laughs] ... So I thought, "Right, lesson learnt, that's why I had to give you this vaccine." [laughs]   *[Anastasia, GP, age 31; Greek]*

Emotional distance not only protected clinical objectivity but also avoided excessive patient dependence on the doctor. However, attaining the right balance was complex. Efforts to minimise distance could threaten to progress too far, causing excessive ownership:

> **ANASTASIA** ... sometimes that's all I did [i.e. walk with the patient]. And just have a chat ... it was a good experience sort of spiritually as well ... The difficulty was ... not knowing where the barriers are; where you are a GP and where you are a friend ... 'cause you sort of ... grieve as well. ... And that [i.e. the patient's death] was a bit difficult, I think. ....   *[Anastasia, GP, age 31; Greek]*

The aim, therefore, in more established or matured doctor–patient relationships often shifted from initial efforts at narrowing distance (as especially emphasised in earlier parts of this chapter), to those of *limiting such a narrowing* or even of *broadening distance*:

ANASTASIA ... it's interesting because, ... not that I've done much more than ... what my job is, [but] ... she's been really grateful about all that [and has said] ... , you know, "Drop in for coffee", ... And ... I think, "No, hang on, is it right for me to sort of drop in for a coffee ... ?", ... you know what I mean? For the barrier ... now all of a sudden the barrier comes down for them and they feel more comfortable about that ... All of a sudden they think, "Oh, you've been through so much with us, so therefore you're no longer our doctor, you're also our friend", sort of thing. ... And then, you know, then they have to come in for pap smears and they have an abnormal pap smear and what do you say to them? ... You know what I mean? So ... it's really hard to sort of ... you know, you don't want to appear like you're offending them but, hey, you know, it's sort of okay [to maintain a bit of a distance] ...

[Anastasia, GP, age 31; Greek]

In such circumstances, patients' usually innocent offerings to the doctor of sweets, home-grown vegetables, or even home-made alcohol (as with Theodore's *[Theodore, GP, age 63; Greek]* patients) could create a considerable moral dilemma for the doctor. Did the acceptance of such offerings imply that the relationship was taking on the social and personal overtones of a friendship? Apart from challenging clinical objectivity, however, a further hazard of 'medical friendships' was their emotional difference from more conventional friendships. Medical friendships could not completely break free of the constraints of the illness and its unpredictability:

BEN ... friendship I think extends the ... doctor–patient relationship. ... I think you can get as close as ... discussing all manner of personal bits and pieces, ... until you get to ... a point where you have to look at the situation [carefully] ... There is a difference with the kind of friendship that tends to develop in ... this kind of relationship ... to ... the majority of your personal friendships, and that difference I think and the dividing line between the two is something that most of us are aware of. If you breach that line you sink your patient, ... and you put unreasonable expectations and demands on them. If you one day ... want the person to ring you and the next day blame them for calling you when ... it's inconvenient, ... you're probably doing no more than many friends would do to each other ... and this would be a thing that the majority of friends' ... situations would get over, but I think the fragility of the circumstances surrounding people in palliative care mitigate against ... too much personal ... exchange, ... too much sharing of warm ... feelings ... and one has to direct the relationship more towards either a counselling function or ... very much a supportive listener.

[Ben, GP, age 49; Jewish]

Generally, the *value* of distance was emphasised more often in GP narratives than in patient and carer narratives. Perhaps this was because the GPs were more acutely aware of the dynamics of the relationship (that is, the professional medical status could not be experienced by patients unless they were medically qualified, whereas doctors had invariably experienced 'patienthood' and might therefore have been more able to differentiate the two). Or perhaps GPs simply had more experience in dealing with terminal illnesses than did patients and families, and such experience had taught them the value of maintaining some distance.

The tension between minimising distance versus avoiding excessive ownership

From the discussion to date, it seems that the mutual coexistence of ownership and distance served to regulate the 'overall' level of distance between doctor and patient. If relationships seemed excessively close, the notion of distance appeared to take on a greater urgency and importance. The opposite occurred in relationships that seemed on the whole to be excessively distant. Attention is here focused on the close relationship, and in particular on *how possible it was* to maintain some distance therein.

Maintaining distance in such a context was generally not easy. Cannon (1989), a sociologist, described the personal and moral struggle involved in such a task regarding her own relationships with her study informants, who were breast cancer patients. The general social prescription for doctor and patient roles usually safeguarded the relationship from gross imbalances in either excessive ownership or distance across professional, social or personal realms. However, two special circumstances created considerable tension in the quest to maintain distance in order to preserve ownership.

The first was when doctor and patient had pre-existing personal or social connections. The medical relationship between Anastasia *[Anastasia, GP, age 31; Greek]* and her mother was an example. There, the emotional distance was so minimal that it prevented medical ownership. Anastasia *[Anastasia, GP, age 31; Greek]* also wondered how well she would cope when the health of her (currently well) older patients would inevitably start to decline. Another dramatic example was provided by Elizabeth, who struggled with professional ownership precisely because social and emotional ownership overwhelmed her sense of professional objectivity and distance:

ELIZABETH ... the second day that I started here, ... a friend of mine who I went to high school with ... brought her daughter in, ... who was five years old, and ...

had been vomiting for three weeks—early morning vomiting only. ... And ... it just set [off] alarm bells straight away, ... so I sent her off for an urgent ... cerebral CT scan, and sure enough she had a ... medulloblastoma, if I recall correctly. ... I had to break that to her ... to *her* [emphasised] ... I mean, I knew her personally, ... the professional aspect had totally gone out of it. ... She was bawling her eyes [out], and believe me, I was bawling my eyes out. ... Two days later the girl lapsed into a coma ... and passed away forty-eight hours later. But ... the emotion ... there was no ... doctor–patient relationship there at all, it was just friend to friend from there on to the end. That was a tragic case, that was awful. ... I still see her, ... she's great now ... she's got four children and ... she's gotten on with her life. ... But ... whenever I see her, I always remember that consultation. ... And ... at times I felt, "Why don't you go to another local doctor?", and initially for the first year or so ... I didn't handle it very well at all, but now we've got a doctor–patient relationship.

[*Elizabeth, GP, age 32; Croatian*]

The second circumstance where it was difficult to maintain an adequate distance was in extremely emotionally charged situations, *irrespective* of how well doctor and patient knew each other. Ben *[Ben, GP, age 49; Jewish]* astutely noted in this regard that '*the gravity of the task tends to be ... mirrored in the strength of the relationships that develop out of it*'. Elizabeth provided an example in her contact with a previously *unknown* patient:

ELIZABETH ... I deliberately try not to [get drawn in emotionally]. ... And I keep saying ... , "Oh ... don't do this. You've got to keep professional, don't show your emotions", but ... sometimes you can't help it. ... I recall an incident, ... wasn't a patient of mine, [she belonged to] one of the other doctors, but he wasn't in so I saw her. ... Her daughter committed suicide ... about two weeks ago, ... and she was re-living the story. I mean, how can you not ... sympathise with this woman? ... And, you know, even though I did not know her, my eyes filled up with tears ...

[*Elizabeth, GP, age 32; Croatian*]

Not surprisingly, the patient-centred approach, more comfortable with minimising distance, was not well adapted to the opposing task of *maintaining* or *enhancing* distance. The emotional nature of such a task meant that it was *not usually possible* to subject such a process to volitional control, as emotion over-rode logical planning and reasoning. The degree of rigidity, therefore, within the doctor and patient roles was variable. That is, doctor and patient roles possessed a certain *fluidity, variability and even an interchangeability* that was emotionally dependent upon the specifics of the illness circumstances. The following sections will examine this interchangeability or reversal of doctor and patient roles. After this, the chapter will conclude with a summary of their implications for medical power.

Role reversal: an introduction

Role reversal extends the discussion of ownership and distance in the doctor–patient relationship. It is concerned not with the overall *magnitude* of ownership or distance (as the preceding sections have already discussed), but rather with its *direction* relative to the doctor and patient role (see Box 4.2).

BOX 4.2 Doctor–patient ownership and distance according to socially prescribed roles

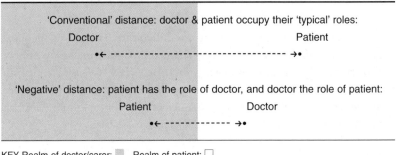

KEY Realm of doctor/carer: ▓ Realm of patient: ☐

The variability in defining the magnitude and direction of distance and ownership between doctors, patients and families implied ambiguity and variability in their roles. Often the doctor became the recipient of care from patients and patients' families, as well as their own family and friends. Patients, in turn, cared for their own carers at home, who themselves did not merely care for the patient but also looked after each other (see Figure 4.1). The potential for role blurring and role reversal was augmented through close interaction under medically and emotionally taxing circumstances.

Role reversal also occurred in contexts outside the immediate doctor–patient relationship. For example, cancer illness in itself dramatically transformed people's lives, altering social, family and work roles, and shaking one's own perception of self. Attention here, however, will focus on the *relationships* between doctor, patient and carer(s). In this setting, specific comment on the concept of role reversal is virtually absent in the medical literature. The closest it gets to the topic is a recognition of excessive ownership (or excessively reduced distance) in the phenomenon

FIGURE 4.1 Direction of care

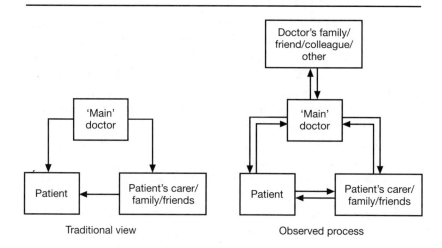

Traditional view   Observed process

of transference and counter-transference in psychotherapy (Gelder, Gath & Mayou, 1986). In general practice writing, Craddock (1976) and McCormick (1979) briefly mention the GP's need to avoid 'transference' (that is, the induction of unwanted psychological dependence in the patient for the doctor), a problem seen to originate in the *patient*. McCormick (1979) considered the GP capable of emotional overdependence on a patient, but the consequences on the dynamics of the relationship and the GP's emotional status were not considered. McWhinney (1989) and McAvoy (1992) recognise the closeness of the GP–patient bond, but do not systematically consider either the potential therapeutic value of such closeness for the person of the doctor, or the potential for role reversal.

The concept of role reversal is perhaps most often discussed in gerontology, where it has also been condemned for its negative portrayal of old age as a 'second childhood' (Brody, 1990). It is also seen in psychological therapy, where it can be incorporated into the technique of 'psychodrama' (O'Driscoll, 1981), or else utilised in the method of 'becoming' the other (Snyder, 1995). In both cases the aim is to enhance the appreciation of the lifeworld of the other and to provide insight into one's own responses to that lifeworld. Discussion on role 'reversal' is also highly developed in Christian theology, centring on the Incarnation of Christ (God becoming man) and the deification of human nature (person becoming God) (Lossky, 1976). Medical role reversal will be described here and reflected against these various writings.

Role reversal: a description

Patients cared for those around them in different ways. Such care was sometimes solicited, and at other times was offered unsolicited. Sometimes the recipients of that care were aware that they were receiving it, and sometimes not. Examples of indirect methods of care included the patient's general demeanour and composure, which helped both the family and the doctor to cope. Maria's *[Maria, age 69 with breast cancer; Peter, age 74—husband; Greek]* acceptance of her illness illustrated this point well—it enabled her to remain calm and practical, thereby assisting her husband to cope. Andrew *[Andrew, GP, age early 40s; Greek]* likewise received valuable indirect support from his patient with advanced prostate cancer, who, during home visits, would want to '*get all his ... medical business out of the way so we could sit down and have a little bit of a talk*' over a piece of cake and some coffee. Maintenance of physical appearance and functional independence likewise assisted the psychological coping of others.

Patients' caring for others was also often manifested more directly. Clare *[Clare, age 65 with stomach cancer; Michael, age 67—husband; Anglo-Celtic]*, for instance, made Michael attend for medical check-ups to ensure that his health would not suffer because of her illness. Concern for the trauma on their families led patients consciously to down-play their symptoms or problems; to consider placing themselves under institutionalised care; or to prefer death if they became too incapacitated and burdensome to their families. (The latter two issues were not observed in Greek–Australian informants.)

Patients' caring for doctors was also very varied. Often it was indirect, such as: maintaining trust and confidence, and not challenging the doctor's authority or knowledge; not taking up doctors' offers to call upon them out of hours; and patiently passing time in the waiting room or at home if the doctor was running late or had mis-scheduled treatment. Often, patients adjusted their approach according to what they perceived the doctor to be feeling:

BEN ... it [i.e. the doctor–patient relationship] is very much a two-way process. ... It's very important for the patient to look after the doctor as well as the doctor to look after the patient. ... And I generally get well looked after. ... I find that ... for those people who are able to, who are mobile, not particularly in any immediate distress, that they're very forgiving towards their doctors, and ... they're very sensitive to ... my moods. ... If I happen to be in a bad one then they'll adjust their requests and their comments accordingly.   *[Ben, GP, age 49; Jewish]*

More direct caring actions also consisted of forgiving doctors for medical mistakes that they were perceived to have made, or of a deep desire to express thanks when the doctor's contribution to the care was seen to be very high:

> **CAROL** ... You don't ever leave ... an Italian or a Greek household without having a cup of tea and some cake or biscuits and all of this sort of stuff [both smile]. And they very often give you gifts ... particularly ... if they have a home garden they always give you gifts and ... it's really very warm ...
>
> *[Carol, GP, age mid-30s; Anglo-Celtic]*

Direct care of doctors was also, however, *practically and medically oriented.* Patients and carers often became skilled in performing medical or nursing tasks as their familiarity of their condition increased. Dimitri *[Barbara, age 48 with cervical cancer; Dimitri, age 53—husband; Greek]*, for instance, administered his wife's subcutaneous calciparine injections daily to prevent venous thrombosis. Others were familiar with managing urinary catheters, attending to basic hygiene needs, or knowing the signs indicating the need for an extra dose of morphine, to cite a few examples. Such expertise could be so developed and astute that it enabled patients themselves to *assist or even train their own doctors in the performance of medical tasks.* An example was seen with a patient regarding the treatment of her malignant skin lesions:

> **BEN** ... over the years I mean she has just picked out the best of the treatments and she knows those sorts of managements that will produce a result. She is ... very, very much into training her doctor and she's trained me in terms of ... how to locally inject her lesions ... and we work together on that, ... experimented in terms of the actual mechanics of it until we got it down to a reasonably fine art.
>
> *[Ben, GP, age 49; Jewish]*

A further example of such medical competence was seen with Simon *[Simon, age 64 with lymphoma; Cynthia, age 52—wife; Anglo-Celtic]*, who could very accurately self-diagnose early tumour recurrences in his skin:

> **CYNTHIA** ... his doctor ... calls him Doctor Simon because he [i.e. Simon] ... finds these lumps and ... he [i.e. Simon's doctor] says, "Is [sic] there any new lumps?", and Simon will say, "Yeah there's one here and there's one there and there's one there", and he [i.e. Simon's doctor] says, "That's right, Doctor Simon" [laughs]
>
> *[Simon, age 64 with lymphoma; Cynthia, age 52—wife; Anglo-Celtic]*

However, such competence and expertise had its stressful aspects. Monica *[Monica, age 48 with breast cancer; Alan, age late 50s—husband; Anglo-Celtic]*, for instance, quickly became aware that a mammogram performed for her inflammatory breast cancer might have facilitated micro-metastatic spread because of the squeezing effect on the breast. That, in turn, introduced tension into the doctor–patient relationship.

Doctors themselves, *irrespective* of whether they performed their medical tasks well, often felt stress and needed moral and emotional support. Sometimes the doctor's anxiety centred on medical uncertainty. In this situation, support and advice from GP and specialist colleagues became invaluable. At other times, the patient's deterioration roused personal sadness and discomfort at the loss and the inability to curtail it. This was often most intense in cases where the patients were either young or where a good prognosis was not realised. Doctors needed care because cancer reminded them of their own mortality:

BEN ... I frequently ... use my colleagues here for debriefing ... and I found that over the last two years, quite a few of them have actually returned the ... compliment and do the same. ... And, and that it's very important for the carer to be cared for, ... both by ... his [sic] patients and by ... you know, from his own personal standpoint, but also must have the assistance and support of his colleagues.

[Ben, GP, age 49; Jewish]

The GP's 'patienthood' before their own patient could be extreme and obvious if the GP was overcome with emotion (recall the examples above provided by Elizabeth *[Elizabeth, GP, age 32; Croatian]*). More often, however, GP patienthood was more subtle; emotions could be revealed in a planned and controlled manner; thereby appearing to 'professionalise', and therefore legitimise, them:

MARGARITA ... but I don't mind emotions at all actually. No, no. ... I accept it as part of my work practice and, and I express it to my patients too. ... I say, "I feel this way", and, and that's okay. ...   *[Margarita, GP, age 33; Greek]*

Often, however, the doctor was the 'silent patient' in the relationship, hiding their difficulties because of their professional sense of duty and their desire not to upset the patient and family. Theodore *[Theodore, GP, age 63; Greek]*, as illustrated earlier, expressed this point concisely and powerfully:

THEODORE ... after you've been around for forty years, a lot of the patients are close. ... In fact I've known them longer than their own children have known them because I can go back four generations. ... I mean ... in forty years it was the great grandmother even. I go sometimes to the cemeteries and have a look at their names and think, "Oh, you know ... there's four or five generations we're talking about. It's been a long time". ... So this closeness is very close and say, you have a bit of a cry for a few seconds and then get back to it. ... I'm allowed to have my emotions. ... I don't cry in front of them. ... No, no I wouldn't do that. They might think they're sicker than they are.

[Theodore, GP, age 63; Greek]

Such difficulties in sharing emotions sometimes extended even to the doctor's family or close colleagues. Recall, for example, the incident described in Chapter 3 involving Carol *[Carol, GP, age mid-30s; Anglo-Celtic]*, who wrote to colleagues interstate about her difficulties:

CAROL ... it wasn't the sort of thing that I could have shared with ... either my partner or ... someone that I work with here ... because I don't think ... they would have understood ... why this situation was stressful.

[Carol, GP, age mid-30s; Anglo-Celtic]

Role reversal: a summary and comparative analysis

From the interview data, seven key features of role reversal in the doctor–patient relationship can be distinguished (see Box 4.3). These are discussed in turn below.

BOX 4.3 Key features of role reversal

Role reversal is distinct from the concepts of ownership and distance.
Role reversal does not obliterate the 'original' role.
Role reversal fluctuates over time and illness circumstances.
Role reversal is not only emotional in its nature, but also 'functional' or practical.
Role reversal can be 'natural' or conflict-based.
Role reversal may be openly manifest or more subtle and hidden.
Role reversal is not merely dyadic but multidimensional.

Role reversal is distinct from the concepts of ownership and distance

Ownership and distance were phenomena that occurred in the context of people remaining *within* their conventional roles: the doctor remained the doctor and the patient remained the patient. This is in keeping with psychoanalytic theory, where transference (a patient projecting emotional issues upon the doctor) and counter-transference (the doctor in turn reacting to such projections) (Gelder et al., 1986) highlight the problem of defining an optimal distance, but frame this problem from the viewpoint of *immovable* roles. Role reversal, however, saw doctor and patient roles as more fluid and not rigidly defined. The patient could care for the doctor in manifold ways, while the doctor could likewise become the care-receiver. The principles of ownership and distance were still valid to those situations, but occurred in the context of reversed roles.

Role reversal does not obliterate the 'original' role

In gerontology, the term 'role reversal' has been criticised because of its potential to belittle ageing as a burdensome process of 'second childhood', ignoring the older person's status of parenthood and personhood (Brody, 1990). Others, however, have noted that ageing undeniably *did* induce dependence in physical tasks (such as feeding, toiletting and basic hygiene) and often in mental and psychological tasks (Berman, 1993). Such authors, therefore, have argued for the phenomenological value of the role reversal concept, provided that it does not imply the loss of original roles.

The data here concurs with such a summation of the concept. Both doctor and patient retained their original roles while *simultaneously* possessing 'opposing' roles of patient and doctor, respectively. The retention of the original role was not an impediment to the existence of genuine role reversal. This is also apparent in autobiographical accounts of doctors who were themselves patients incapacitated by cancer: their medical role remained highly operative despite their patienthood (see Vanderwoude, 1988). This was apparent in their independent summation of their condition, their advice and suggestions for management, and their speculation on their prognostic outlook.

The firm retention of one's original role denotes that this experience is slightly different to that induced by the psychological technique of 'becoming' the other (Snyder, 1995). There, one can 'bypass' transference and counter-transference reactions because 'both persons are simultaneously (immersed) in(to) the same experiential world' (Snyder, 1995), implying a sense of role *convergence* or *merging*, which differs from the phenomenon here described. Role convergence also differs from the Christian notion of deification, where perfect union between a person and God does not subsume or overwhelm one's unique personhood and identity, which remains intact (Lossky, 1976).

Role reversal fluctuates over time and illness circumstances

The dynamic nature of palliative care and the continually changing illness circumstances saw the processes of ownership, distance and role reversal as not rigid, but rather as being fluid or fluctuant over time. Theodore *[Theodore, GP, age 63; Greek]* had '*been crying over one cancer patient for the last ten bloody years*' but such sorrow was intermittent because the patient outlived her medical prognosis despite having a '*massive cancer on her lungs*'. In the same sentence, therefore, Theodore said that '*she's still alive and well … and she feels fit as a fiddle apart from the cough*' *[Theodore, GP, age 63; Greek]*.

Role fluctuation induced by *present* circumstances was not completely independent of *previous* events or experiences in the illness. Rather, these shaped current illness situations and therefore influenced the nature of role fluctuation. Monica *[Monica, age 48 with breast cancer; Alan, age late 50s—husband; Anglo-Celtic]*, for example, finding that she could not continue working whilst having chemotherapy, was forced to retire. She subsequently accepted the patient role more fully and also 'regrouped', becoming more influential in caring for her own family carers.

Role reversal is not only emotional in nature, but also 'functional' or practical

The nature of the role reversal was not located purely in the emotional realm. Rather, it was also located on a practical level that conveyed true qualities of the doctor role to patients, and the patient role to doctors. Ben's *[Ben, GP, age 49; Jewish]* patient, for instance, taught him how to inject her skin lesions, and Simon *[Simon, age 64 with lymphoma; Cynthia, age 52—wife; Anglo-Celtic]* directed his doctor's attention to new clinical signs. Doctors likewise often adopted true characteristics of the patient role. Such characteristics were often a reaction to the situation as it belonged to another, although cancer also physically belonged to the self in terms of one's own potential vulnerability. Doctors often shared their frustrations and sadness with patients (that is, they externalised their own patient role) but more often relied on their own family for support, particularly their spouses.

Role reversal can be natural or conflict-based

Role reversal was often a phenomenon that evolved *naturally*, as relationships and familiarity between doctor, patient and carer matured. Natural role reversal was facilitated by a close sense of ownership, and also by challenging circumstances where emotional release could not be held back. Sometimes, however, role reversal was conflict-based and therefore forced and unnatural. There, mutual consensus (or at least mutual appreciation and understanding) of the other's role in relation to one's own was lacking. The phenomenon of role-forcing of doctors (Glaser & Strauss, 1965) was an example of conflict-based role reversal: in attempting to optimise a medical performance perceived as incompetent or substandard, patients and carers themselves inadvertently assumed the medical role. Often, the silent, ominous, 'background' presence of medico-legal retribution assumed the function of role-forcing on the behalf of patients and carers. This was especially strong if familiarity or comfort between doctor and patient were low. The presence of a medical hierarchy also potentially facilitated role-forcing if GPs were seen to be lacking relative to the specialists.

In more stable and familiar relationships, however, the medico-legal threat gave way to ownership and to natural role reversal. Each party was secure that the other was actively willing and trying to assist them. This completely dismantled any notion of role-forcing, even in situations where the patient had technically to direct the GP in their medical task. Ben *[Ben, GP, age 49; Jewish]* was not embarrassed that his patient had to train him to inject her skin lesions, nor did it seem unnatural or unusual to the patient that she had to do so. Without obliterating the distinction between doctor and patient, ownership paradoxically facilitated a context of true partnership where role reversal was a *natural accompaniment*. It was precisely in this context that medical uncertainty also posed less threat to the relationship, itself becoming a more natural and expected part of the illness that would be negotiated by doctor, patient and family in partnership.

Role reversal may be openly manifest or more subtle and hidden

The degree to which role reversal was outwardly manifest was variable. Patients' efforts to care for their doctors were often subtle and well camouflaged, but could also be more openly manifest. The motivation for such efforts was usually *not*, in the primary instance, an awareness that the doctor *needed* to be cared for. Rather, it stemmed from a sense of ownership that made patients *want* to care for their doctors. The extension of themselves to incorporate the caring role for their own doctors and carers was thus a 'natural' outcome (as discussed above) that was also *self-therapeutic*, imparting a sense of purpose, achievement and contentment. The extent to which doctors revealed their own acceptance, need and appreciation of such care was also variable.

The subtlety of role reversal as detected here contrasts to the more concrete examples induced in the psychological exercise of psychodrama. There, 'reversal' is more obvious and complete, but also at the same time more artificial and short lived, lasting the mere duration of the session.

Role reversal is not merely dyadic but multidimensional

Giving and receiving care were complex social issues that were often not clearly distinguishable. For example, even simple actions, such as complying with medical instructions to take a drug, could be seen as a form of active care for the doctor. A key question, therefore, is what imparts to an action the quality of caring for *other* in addition to caring for *self*? The answer lay in the notion of ownership, which dissolved the formality with which care is typically conceptualised, especially its rigid sense of *direction* based on socially defined roles (that is, the idea that a doctor *gives* care and a patient *receives* it).

The *dissolution of direction* in the notion of care not only made role reversal a natural phenomenon, freeing it from the formalities and constraints imposed by such direction, but also imparted *multidimensional qualities* to it. Role reversal therefore did not *only* apply to or incorporate doctor and patient roles (which have formed the focus of the present discussion), but caring and receiving care *simultaneously* occurred along many other dimensions. The doctor, for instance, could be doctor, patient, carer, friend and relative to both the patient and the patient's carer; they, in turn, could be likewise to each other, as well as to the doctor. Such a synthesis differs from the more dyadic nature of role reversal as it has been discussed in gerontology, which focuses only on the parent–child dimension in terms of dependence versus independence.

Distance, ownership and role reversal, and implications for medical power

The dynamic interplay between ownership and distance, and the nature and existence of role reversal in medical practice have been presented as new concepts. By providing additional insight on the nature of medical power and the doctor–patient relationship, these concepts hold significant implications for clinical practice as advocated by the patient-centred approach. This chapter concludes by summarising these key issues.

Distance, ownership and compatibility: bridging observed paradoxes

Against the ultimate goal of effectively managing ill health, the central and ongoing task of each illness participant was to optimise ownership and distance in their relationships with others. This central task set the background against which issues of compatibility and medical uncertainty were realised and contextualised. It offered a theoretical foundation from which to unify and explain two key paradoxes in medical relationships that defied the predictions of the patient-centred approach.

The first of these paradoxes was the existence of a good doctor–patient compatibility in the face of much uncertainty and physical and emotional adversity caused by the illness, even in the relative *absence* of patient-centredness. Recall, for example, Jane's [*Jane, English, age 61 with mycosis fungoides; John, German, age 70—husband*] good relationship with her disease-oriented dermatologist (p. 36). Here, elements of ownership that paradoxically coexisted with distance were able to predominate and hold the relationship together.

The second of these paradoxes was the lack of compatibility between doctor and patient in circumstances which faced relatively less uncertainty and illness-related adversity, *despite* the application of the patient-centred approach. Recall, for instance, the incident between Andrew [*Andrew, GP, age early 40s; Greek*], a highly patient-centred doctor, and his patient on the issue of prostate cancer screening (p. 130).

Here, elements of distance disrupted a comfortable sense of ownership between doctor and patient.

Bridging distance to facilitate ownership was often a main requirement in relatively new doctor–patient relationships. The opposite task of *maintaining* or even *broadening* distance in order to prevent excessive ownership became increasingly necessary in more established and close doctor–patient relationships. The emotive circumstances of the illness, however, often meant that excessive ownership was hard to avoid, and so the very distinctiveness of doctor, patient and carer roles became blurred and less well defined. It seemed that all, equally, were victims of the cancer illness.

In this light, the adage of treating patient and family as a whole is opened to complete reinterpretation if the response to the crucial question 'Who is family?' (Aldridge, 1987) includes the GP him or herself. In the specific context of the clinical encounter, therefore, medical power is 'humanised' or 'personalised', revealing vulnerabilities and dilemmas as well as strengths. This 'human face' of medical power stands in contrast to accusations labelling it a suppressive, domineering or oppressive force used to maintain class dominance (see Willis, 1983). Here, it was mutual ownership, and *not* dominance, that justified the acceptability of the term 'patient' to all of the study informants, as also implied by Stevens (1994): 'If you call my customers "patients", I shall give them what they need; "clients", what they pay for; "consumers", what they want.'

Role reversal: destructive or therapeutic?

It was shown that a close sense of ownership between doctor and patient was a prime factor that could blur their socially sanctioned roles and set up the possibility of role reversal. This phenomenon, however, did not obliterate one's original role, but simultaneously *coexisted* with it. Although seemingly antithetical at first sight, the coexistence of 'carer' and 'care-receiver' roles represented a *natural progression* in the relationship, reflecting human needs within it. 'Natural' role and 'reversed' role existed concurrently and naturally (or automatically), sometimes without sharp distinction and often *without a conscious awareness* of their enactment or presence.

The important implication for medical power was that giving care and receiving care were not mutually exclusive. This contradicts the strong sense of *direction* implied in the term 'care', which has influentially shaped (and restricted) the manner in which the doctor–patient relationship has been conceived. According to the evidence presented, role reversal in functionally stable relationships was an *integral and necessary* part of the therapeutic relationship that itself *contributed* to the therapeutic effects for both doctor and patient. It was integral because it was intimately entwined with human emotion, which was not always subject to absolute control through rational volition. It was therapeutic in the sense of fulfilling the patient's need to care for others, and the doctor's need to be cared for. In that sense, role reversal was as much a moral issue as it was a practical one. People *wanted care* and *wanted to care.*'

Broad reflections on medical power and the patient-centred approach

General practice texts make much of patient-centredness, itself strengthened through continuity of care. However, they do not adequately emphasise the limits to which such patient-centredness can be taken. Because they characterise patient-centredness according to a well-defined sense of professional distance, problems of excessive ownership and role reversal are barely considered. The potential for both excessive distance and excessive ownership is more inherent in the emotionally difficult and challenging situations described in the palliative care literature. However, even this body of writing is not clearly framed in terms of the coexistence of ownership and distance, and the potential for role reversal.

The notions of ownership, distance and role reversal demand a critical review of the patient-centred method. Very broadly, the socio-historical evolution of this method (described in the Introduction) was based on the existence of a gulf or distance between doctor and patient that had to be bridged (recall that scientific biomedicine had negated the social presence of the patient). This detracted emphasis from the necessity of *maintaining* some distance, and from the potential for excessive ownership and role reversal. The patient-centred method can too easily blame doctors for 'rocky' relationships. Such accusations stem not only from external sources, but also potentially from within the very doctor themselves (Dozor & Addison, 1992). Patient-centredness in this context has positivist overtones in implying that relationships can be readily optimised if the doctor follows a few prescribed rules (while these 'ground-rules' are important, they cannot guarantee success). This is also the sense in the theorising of an ideal medical 'caring role' (Still & Todd, 1986), which fails to consider the context of interaction by problematically implying that a given doctor *uniformly and consistently* either possesses it or does not possess it. A true patient centredness must instead be interactive and consider how the unique context and circumstances shape the clinical relationship. There are no hard and fast rules in palliative care, only principles. Medical education in this field, stressing principles and not rules, merely prepares the doctor for challenges that can only be fully defined within the context of the individual encounter. The individual GP informants did not behave uniformly, but differently according to the case at hand, as do all doctors. Specific actions had to be interpreted according to their context. Medical 'withdrawal', for instance, was sometimes reactive and not voluntary or malicious; conversely, it could be voluntary and deliberate to the benefit of all if it curbed excessive ownership.

The patient-centredness of the doctor ultimately cannot be properly viewed apart from the doctor-centredness of the patient and family. Suggestions that doctors have rights to terminate the therapeutic relationship *for the sake of the patient* in the event of irreconcilable differences between them (Siegler, 1981) silently attest to this. Such suggestions are rare in medical and sociological writing, where termination of medical relationships is usually described as patient-initiated in response to medical ineptitude or insensitivity.

Conclusion: towards a new model of the clinical encounter

All of the preceding discussion has suggested a notion of medical power as simultaneously vulnerable while remaining strong, simultaneously uncertain while remaining certain, and simultaneously lacking control while possessing control. It has shown that both 'illness' and 'disease' as defined by Kleinman (1978) and distinguished in the patient-centred approach of McWhinney (1989) (see Introduction, Boxes I.7 and I.8) were *not* independent and isolated topics, but *inseparable* problems that had to be met concurrently. The distinction between 'caring' for the 'illness' versus 'curing' the 'disease' (Kleinman, 1978) did not offer any real insight into the unique dynamics of the clinical encounter. Rather, it was the interplay between ownership and distance, and the existence of role reversal that opened up insight into the nature and accessibility of this complex field. Importantly, these concepts have also shown that 'care' did not imply the strong sense of *direction* (that is, *from* doctor *to* patient) that is assumed in medical and sociological writing.

The final chapter will begin by briefly overviewing the nature of medical power according to the conclusions reached in these discussion chapters, specifically addressing the research problems posed in the Introduction. This forms a foundation on which a new model of GP–cancer patient interaction in palliative care is presented: the Model of Bi-Directional Care.

Bi-directional care between doctor and patient: a new model

The first part of this chapter uses the conclusions of the preceding chapters to systematically address the key questions and problems posed about medical power in the Introduction (these are summarised in Box 5.1). The second part of the chapter then employs this analysis as a foundation to develop and discuss a new model of GP–cancer patient interaction, the Model of Bi-Directional Care. This model will be compared with and contrasted against the Patient-Centred Method (Introduction, Box I.8), currently the 'gold-standard' family medicine model, to generate new perspectives in the understanding of medical power and the doctor–patient relationship.

BOX 5.1 Key unanswered issues in medical power

The level of 'patient-centredness' within the patient-centred approach
The differing forms of medical power
The influence of medical power upon the medical profession itself
The relationship between medical power and moral or ethical issues
Circumstances, methods and consequences of challenges to medical power
The permanence or reversibility of medical power

The nature and quality of medical power: a summary

The notion that medical power is a largely negative, dominating force is an unbalanced one that has confused its function, place and influence in the clinical setting. Medical power is a complex phenomenon that is both framed and expressed according to broad social and cultural norms beyond the individual control of either doctor or patient, as well as particular factors *within* the personal interaction between these persons. The key questions posed of medical power in the Introduction related to how it was defined, experienced and refined over time within the context of the doctor–patient–family relationship. These questions are addressed below.

The level of 'patient-centredness' of the patient-centred approach

The *intent* of the doctor in their practice of medicine is a factor not emphasised enough in sociological and medical literature. A pessimistic view might interpret 'patient-centredness' as a mere tool or strategy that can be mechanically or dispassionately applied by the doctor in order to gain cooperation, and therefore control, in the consultation. Fortunately, according to the findings here, this was not generally so. Cooperation was not sought because of a medical desire to control, but rather of a desire to personalise and 'humanise' the process of care.

The notions of ownership and distance, however, showed that even such genuine and sincere intent could vary in terms of the emotional investment that it extracted from the doctor. The distinction between the 'main doctor' versus the 'temporary doctor' illustrated the point well: although both could be perfectly patient-centred, it was the 'main' doctor, the doctor closest to the patient, who was prone to be more emotionally subjective in their execution of care.

Role reversal added a further dimension by showing that the origin of a genuine patient-centred approach did not centre exclusively upon the doctor, but depended heavily upon the dynamics of doctor–patient interaction. Role reversal could paradoxically facilitate the execution of patient-centredness, in that the doctor's vulnerability and uncertainty offered a unique opportunity to satisfy the fundamental need of patients to be able to give, that is, to offer care to others. Role reversal in this sense solidified the patient's sense of self-worth and simultaneously buoyed medical power itself by demonstrating its acceptance of its limitations. Indeed, the notion of 'medical power' was foreign and no longer existent in such relationships—it had been obliterated and was superseded by the closeness of the relationship itself. As a natural phenomenon (Chapter 4, p. 152), role reversal was the ultimate expression of the 're-humanisation' of the clinical encounter.

This view of the doctor–patient relationship is in contrast to the literature on the patient-centred approach and related models (see the Introduction, Boxes I.7, I.8). These tend to implicate the doctor as the determining source of the success of the approaches, without adequately considering broader factors impinging on the dynamics of the individual relationship. The generalised notion of a medical 'ideal type' (Still & Todd, 1986) was also flawed on this very point: a doctor demonstrating caring qualities in terminal illness was seen as a uniform type that would *consistently* perform in like manner across *every* terminal illness situation that confronted them. Quite the opposite was suggested by the informants of this study: the dynamics of the particular interaction harboured its strength (or weakness), and the uniqueness of each relationship and situation was not as readily or confidently translatable to other relationships and situations.

The differing forms of medical power

Medical power could be both desirable, as in its ability to alleviate symptoms, as well as undesirable, as in its potential to emphasise the disease rather than the individual. Its expression could also be highly variable, ranging from forceful and obvious to subtle and almost imperceptible.

The form that medical power took depended upon how and where the notion of power itself was constructed. It was shown in Chapter 2 that medical power was located not only within the body of medicine as a whole, but also within the individual doctor, through whom it had to be channelled, as well as in the patient and the patient's family, who ultimately had to sanction the operation of this power upon themselves, yielding themselves to it. Such sanctioning involved a process whereby pre-existing and often abstract views of medical power, formed when people are healthy and influenced by general social opinion, had to be reconciled with their lived experience of serious illness. Finally, the particular course of the illness, often roughly predictable but essentially unforeseeable, also influenced medical power. Unexpected circumstances located beyond medical control, either positive or negative, respectively either bolstered or degraded the perception of medical power by patient or family. So medical power was also, in a certain sense, located within the realm of *chance*.

Ultimately, the effectiveness of medical power was not determined by the *absolute* quality or type of expression that it adopted, but rather by the *degree to which doctor and patient concurred on such an expression.* This determined whether therapy was interpreted as 'active' or 'passive', and also shaped the nature and definition of uncertainty itself.

Finally, a sense of ownership between doctor and patient could facilitate and bolster medical power even in its admission of uncertainty and its inability to cure. Role reversal went a step further in demonstrating the vulnerability of medicine through the individual doctor. This vulnerability again, however, paradoxically *bolstered* medical power through allowing it to receive assistance in order to continue being effective in its own task of healing (rather than curing).

The influence of medical power upon the medical profession itself

Pressure on doctors to perform to high standards emanated not only from the general public but also from *within* the profession itself. Such pressure, a form of role-forcing, could be asymmetrical (as when hierarchical authority was exerted) or symmetrical (as in the expectations that colleagues of equal medical 'rank' had of each other) (see Groopman, 1987; Bosk, 1979). The role of the individual doctor therefore incorporated professional as well as public expectations; expectations which committed doctors themselves accepted and aspired to meet.

Such ideals, however, rested uneasily against the reality of ubiquitous and variable forms of clinical uncertainty that faced the doctor, against which the body of medicine had few satisfactory solutions. It was only the sense of ownership between doctor and patient that was ultimately capable of removing the direction or responsibility towards responding to uncertainty. That is, uncertainty (and even medical mistakes) were no longer exclusively the doctor's, but rather also belonged to the patient and their family as a whole. Medically irresolvable uncertainty was thus transformed and made potentially capable of being solved when viewed in such a different and collective context. Role reversal, as a culmination of ownership, went further by potentially placing much of the responsibility to respond to uncertainty with the patient or their carers.

Medicine's failure hitherto to formally describe such phenomena does not necessarily imply that it has been blinded by its own striving and desire for control and high standards of care. It may rather indicate that the processes of ownership and of role reversal, as observed here, were often *subtle*. This subtlety meant that they could be easily overlooked because they were often enacted *unconsciously and automatically* at the individual level by both doctor and patient alike. These centrally important intricacies in doctor–patient encounters, and their relevance to doctor–patient harmony, need to become more fully crystallised into the academic consciousness of medicine.

The relationship between medical power and moral or ethical issues

The ethical issues that most frequently challenged and threatened medical power were often subtle and related to the more 'everyday' and 'routine' aspects of interpersonal interaction, rather than to highly specific and relatively far less frequent issues such as euthanasia.

The Introduction and Chapter 3 illustrated how progressive biomedical sophistication in medicine *generated* moral or ethical dilemmas in clinical management. This occurred not only through obliterating the social standing of the patient and emphasising curing above healing, but also by raising questions about the suitability, applicability, safety, cost and accessibility of diagnostic and therapeutic methods.

Attempts to rediscover the social presence of the patient, however, also generated their own specific moral and ethical problems. For example, the patient-centred approach demanded efforts at doctor–patient cooperation, but offered no practical solutions if such efforts failed. On varying issues, it was seen that both GPs as well as patients and their carers had personal limits beyond which they could not travel in their attempts to compromise or negotiate.

True compromise and negotiation also presumed that the issue at hand was *clearly and uniformly* understood by all parties. However, the inherent limitations of spoken language, the inability to live the precise emotional experience of the other, the difference in medical knowledge between doctor, patient and family, as well as the inherently different vantage point of each person involved with the illness all indicated that even major issues and tasks in the illness were not understood by each party in a uniform or compatible manner. Therefore, even the seemingly simple and 'obvious' medical ethical principle of full disclosure and informed consent could be potentially destructive and harmful if not concordant to the thinking of patients and families. Ultimately, it was only within the dynamics of the clinical encounter that moral issues could be properly contextualised. Outside this context, blanket rules such as full disclosure and informed consent were effectively rendered meaningless.

Moral uncertainty was also linked to an improper balance of ownership and distance within the professional relationship. The patient-centred method encouraged a narrowing of distance between doctor and patient but did not necessarily safeguard it from the dilemmas of *excessive* reduction of distance (that is, excessive ownership), which might compromise medical objectivity. The need to maintain or enhance distance to prevent excessive ownership was often a moral necessity but was simultaneously challenging because of the strength of the emotional bond between doctor and patient that had, by that time, developed.

Often, however, the *coexistence* of ownership with distance kept the relationship appropriately balanced. The natural and often unconscious phenomenon of role reversal created moral and ethical paradoxes in that it made the care of the doctor a *legitimate* task that did not compromise the care of the patient, but rather *enhanced* it through imparting to them a sense of meaning and purpose.

Circumstances, methods and consequences of challenges to medical power

Medical power was challenged by patients and families in different ways, ranging from implicit (such as non-compliance or gentle questioning of medical actions) to explicit (such as abandoning or criticising the doctor). The discrepancy between the *actual* versus the *perceived* potential of medical power also contributed to such challenges. This was evident, for example, in patients' questioning and perplexity as to why medical tests might have initially failed to reveal the diagnosis of cancer or its complications. Such challenges could be directed to the individual GP, or could be aimed more broadly at the medical profession in general, depending on the individual circumstances.

GPs themselves also challenged medical power particularly in regard to its tendency to drift away from patient-centredness. It is in this regard that the use of clinical 'rules' or protocols (such as the need for universal, open disclosure) could be seen as inconsiderate of the unique circumstances of each case. Another method of challenge utilised by GPs was their open admission of clinical uncertainty and their attempts to bridle the often excessively high hopes that medicine sometimes generated in patients and families. This was especially so in cancer illness, where patients might be exposed to complex and impressive technological gadgetry and instrumentation that might trigger excessive hopes for cure.

The key issue for the doctor–patient relationship, however, was not *whether* medical power was challenged, but *how* it was challenged. The inevitability of some form of challenge rested in medicine's inability to cure most forms of cancer. In circumstances where an overall sense of ownership prevailed between doctor and patient, challenges to medical authority and power were often directed to the broader fraternity of medicine (for example, its inability to cure, the nasty side effects of its medications and treatments, its diagnostic limitations, and so on), *without* denigrating the person of the doctor for belonging to such a fraternity. In those circumstances, challenges were 'friendly', being either inquisitive or else an expression of frustration in the limitations of medicine, which, importantly, were *accepted* by the patient. This form of challenge to medical power actually assisted the therapeutic process by assuring that the therapeutic direction was realistically focused. Interestingly, in such close doctor–patient relationships, role reversal itself, often occurring naturally or subconsciously, was not a threat or a challenge to medical power. It was not a phenomenon that highlighted medicine's weakness, but rather a phenomenon that revealed medicine's human face.

In situations where there was an excessive distance between doctor and patient, challenges to medical power were often more directed to the person of the GP as the responsible representative of the entire medical profession, and such challenges had the potential to be more aggressive. Sometimes these challenges varied a little by targeting the GP entirely, rather than additionally implicating the entire medical profession through them. In those cases, role-forcing (Glaser & Strauss, 1965) was often observed and the relationship was often an unhappy one. Although such challenges might have been justifiable in that the individual doctor's performance was poor, they also often stemmed from a *non-acceptance* of the incurability or progression of the illness on the part of patient and/or family.

The permanence or reversibility of medical power

The manner of progression through the illness (in terms of its biological course and the interactions centred around managing it) had the potential to alter the status or the nature of medical power. For instance, complications arising from therapy might see medical power progress from being respected to being criticised. Other situations, such as unexpectedly good progress, might see the converse, with medical power increasing from being initially criticised to being finally appreciated.

Chapter 2 also showed that progression through the illness was often at the mercy of circumstances completely external to the clinical interaction itself. This was the realm of chance, where the unexpectedly sudden relapse or deterioration, the unpredictable but severe adverse reaction to a medicine, or the acutely destructive and psychologically devastating illness complication belonged. At times, such uncontrollable factors could also be positive, such as an unexpectedly *good* response to therapy, and so on.

Although relevant in shaping the form and nature of medical power, the *permanence* or *reversibility* of events in the illness could only be properly understood or contextualised against the notions of ownership and distance. This held true irrespective of whether such events were positive or negative, expected or unexpected, frequent or infrequent, or whether they resulted from the therapeutic interaction or were completely determined by chance.

In situations of optimal ownership (characterised by an appropriately minimal distance between doctor and patient), negative events or circumstances seemed relatively less permanent in their effects upon the relationship and upon the general standing of medicine in the eyes of the patient. Positive events or factors in this setting were magnified and took on a greater sense of permanency, imparting to the relationship and to medical power a greater sense of solidity and stability.

Conversely, in the setting of excessive distance between doctor and patient, negative events or circumstances made a more permanent impact that obstinately reverberated throughout the remaining course of the illness. Likewise, in this setting, positive events or circumstances were more likely to be less influential in upholding medical power. The key (as Chapter 2 concluded) was to optimise the relationship *early* and hope that fortune (in the form of uncontrollably negative illness progress) would not undo such efforts. Once a foundation was present, relationships generally held more secure and stable against the buffeting of negative progress.

In the phenomenon of role reversal, even though the doctor was receiving care in addition to providing it, the standing of medicine and medical power itself was not compromised. Instead, it was paradoxically strengthened through the individual doctor's human responses to the illness, providing the patient and family with an opportunity to care for the doctor which in turn facilitated the doctor's ongoing care of them.

Bi-Directional Care: a model of GP–patient interaction in palliative care

Having summarised the key findings relating to medical power, attention is now turned towards using them to construct a new model of GP–cancer patient interaction, the Model of Bi-Directional Care. A consequence of this process will be a critical re-evaluation of the patient-centred model (McWhinney, 1989, Figure 5.1), which currently represents family medicine's 'gold-standard' approach (see the Introduction for a discussion of the socio-historical evolution of this model).

FIGURE 5.1 The patient-centred clinical method

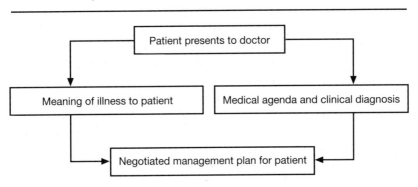

The models are distinguished in their essence by one important facet: the patient centred model, although to a degree *descriptive* of good or 'healthy' doctor–patient relationships, is largely *prescriptive*. That is, it is largely a *method*, a clinical tool that can be consciously *applied* by the doctor to optimise their working relationship with the patient. The Model of Bi-Directional Care, conversely, is more *descriptive* rather than *prescriptive*; it is effectively a representation of the *consequences* of the patient-centred method. It also more particularly deals with doctor–patient interactions characterised by a lasting presence of *harmony*. This will become more apparent as the model itself is systematically constructed and discussed in the following sub-sections.

Bi-Directional Care: foundations

Given that the Model of Bi-Directional Care is largely descriptive of the consequences of the patient-centred method, its foundations are relatively similar (Figure 5.2).

FIGURE 5.2 Bi-Directional Care: foundations

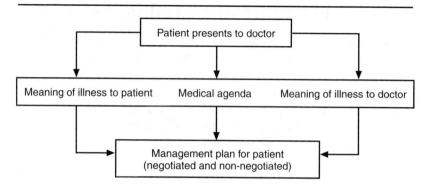

The patient presents (or is presented to) the doctor with an initial clinical problem, which subsequent interaction aims to alleviate or resolve. In this interaction, as in the patient–centred model, account is taken of the highly variable (and not necessarily negative) meaning of the illness to the patient and their family, as described in Chapter 1. Such illness meaning had to be harmonised with the medical agenda at hand, itself founded on scientific knowledge about the pathophysiology and management of disease. Pre-existing familiarity between doctor and patient through previous clinical encounters assisted the task of harmonisation through discussion and negotiation.

Chapter 1, however, also demonstrated that cancer illness had significant emotional and psychological meaning for the doctor. It identified six particular ways of viewing or 'feeling' the clinical situation, with emphasis on 'epidemiological', 'disease burden', 'functional', 'intuitive', 'chronicity' and 'partnership' factors (see p. 46–60). These different emphases affected the way that even concrete or 'clear-cut' medical agendas were understood and executed. Well-defined and supposedly unambiguous protocols were therefore subjected to a certain *flexibility* in terms of how doctors understood them, emotionally reacted to them, and delivered them.

It is this latter dimension, the meaning of the illness to the doctor, and the particular 'flavour' that it imparted to the management process, that is relatively underdeveloped in general practice texts on the doctor–patient relationship. Not surprisingly, it is completely missing from largely patient-oriented accounts of general practice, such as Stimson & Webb (1975). More surprisingly, however, GP-authored texts such as Morrell (1976) and Murtagh (1994) do not specifically discuss it, while others highlight it to varying degrees. Browne & Freeling (1976: 14–19) outlined the importance of the 'emotional experience evoked in the examining doctor by the attitude and bearing of the patient', and how that enhanced the doctor's understanding of the patient. However, with the exception of McWhinney (1989: 80–5), who clearly acknowledged that such personal feelings are inherent *within* the doctor, making 'detached objectivity' essentially impossible, other texts emphasise a more *external* origin of such feelings. This effectively equated such feelings to 'counter-transference', implying that they were a secondary or reactive response by the doctor to the actions and responses of the patient (see Browne & Freeling, 1976; McAvoy, 1992; Craddock, 1976; and McCormick, 1979). No emphasis was placed on the pre-existing feelings and attitudes within the doctor (reflecting their personality and clinical experience), feelings that themselves determined the nature of the 'counter-transference' response. Furthermore, Chapter 2 showed the dynamic inter-relationship between the meaning of the illness for the patient, the medical agenda and the meaning of the illness for the doctor. These three components are therefore represented within a single box in Figure 5.2. This fed into the generation of a management plan.

Unlike the idealised goal of the patient-centred method of McWhinney (1989), the management plan shown in Figure 5.2 was not entirely based on 'pure' negotiation. 'Negotiation' as understood by general practice texts rests upon the intimate knowledge that a GP gains of 'their' patients over time and with repeated contact. Negotiation, as shown by Chapter 2, therefore began from predetermined starting points which seemed reasonable, and not completely *de novo*. Indeed, this also occurred in first-ever encounters where doctor and patient were unfamiliar to each other, because of the gap in clinical knowledge between them. This required the translation of complex biomedical information into everyday language, but the content, detail and clarity of such a translation remained largely at the discretion of the doctor. Disclosure of diagnosis, as discussed in Chapter 2, for instance, was not a binomial issue of 'knowing' versus 'not knowing', or 'telling' versus 'not telling', but represented a potential spectrum of awareness and telling. Patients and their families, in their turn, also guided the direction of negotiation by being at times selective in what they would share with the doctor, emotionally and otherwise.

It was such an understanding of negotiation as a relative phenomenon that explained why it was not always welcomed. Doctors sometimes skewed information to support their own particular view of management. Patients, likewise, sometimes found negotiation and their involvement in clinical decision making uncomfortable, relegating all decision-making to the doctors. The only negotiation in such cases was that there should be explanation but *no* negotiation as such! It is important to note that such situations, when founded upon mutual understanding and trust, actually *stemmed* from a harmonious doctor–patient relationship, rather than threatening it or being incompatible with it. The precise nature of such a harmony was to be understood in the context of a continuing care, where time and the dynamically evolving interplay between ownership and distance shaped the relationship and, through it, the interpretation and nature of uncertainty itself. Attention is now turned to these issues.

Bi-Directional Care: effects of uncertainty and continuity of care

Time changed people and changed the nature of the doctor–patient relationship (Figure 5.3).

FIGURE 5.3 Bi-Directional Care: effects of continuity

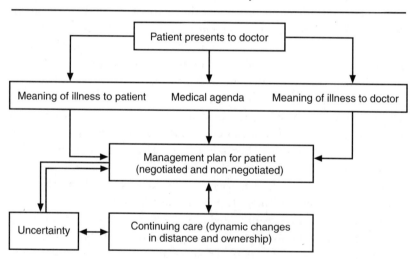

Cancer's complexity, its relatively rapid evolution and its emotional impacts on patients and families required a regular process of medical monitoring. Such frequent doctor–patient contact in the face of progressive disease and impending death added emotional and spiritual dimensions to the nature of that relationship that made it quite different to that of ordinary clinical contacts. Such continuity of care highlighted the dynamic interplay in the levels of perceived ownership and distance that doctor and patient felt towards each other. It therefore appears in Figure 5.3 as a distinct category, a temporal extension of the management plan for the patient, from which it stemmed and which it, in turn, affected.

Chapter 4, in particular, showed that while the early task within a relationship was to minimise distance, later tasks were often oriented around maintaining or even enhancing distance. This was due to the emotional impacts of the illness trajectory upon the doctor in terms of their own personal vulnerability, as well as their distress for the patient's suffering in its own right. This point was recognised by McWhinney (1989), who wrote of the delicate balance between appropriate and inappropriate attachment:

> The behaviour expected of physicians has been detached objectivity … I do not think that family physicians have ever practised in this way. For one thing, one cannot enter into long-term relations with people without affections developing, and it is inevitable that these affections will show. … It is important, however, to distinguish between this closeness and the kind of emotional attachment that satisfies the physician's personal needs. To avoid the pitfall of filling our own emotional needs through the doctor–patient relationship requires self-knowledge.
>
> (McWhinney, 1989: 84)

What was not clearly apparent in McWhinney's (1989) writing was the intricate and dynamic coexistence, inter-relationship and inter-dependence between distance and ownership in the doctor–patient relationship (as outlined in Chapter 4). This absence made the dividing line between 'appropriate' closeness versus 'inappropriate' closeness seem relatively clear cut, which contradicted the complex and often subtle nature of the emotional and moral uncertainty seen here in the narrative accounts of GPs, patients and carers (as seen in Chapter 3).

Uncertainty itself makes a distinct appearance in Figure 5.3. Uncertainty in general was a major and universal threat to the stability of the management plan, the composure of doctor and patient and the stability of the doctor–patient relationship. Chapter 3 discussed the different components of uncertainty, which included knowledge-related uncertainty, uncertainty related to health-care structure, process-related uncertainty, inherent medical uncertainty, uncertainty in the negotiation of different paradigms of illness, and moral and emotional uncertainty.

Uncertainty, although an important *influence* on doctor–patient harmony and compatibility in initial management and continuing care, was itself, in turn, *affected* by these (hence the bilateral direction of the arrows in Figure 5.3). Chapter 3 has shown, for instance, that a good, mutual understanding between doctor and patient of each other's predicament might nullify the tension associated with uncertainty. Such a relationship, however, could also make uncertainty harder to bear because of the heightened sense of loss that it could engender in both doctor and patient. Conversely, in situations where doctor–patient harmony was poor, uncertainty could enhance such instability. Such instability, in turn, could further magnify the presence of uncertainty and more negatively influence the emotional perception of it.

It was therefore time and the nature of the consolidating union between doctor and patient that contextualised uncertainty. Chapters 2 and 3 showed that the distinction between 'active' treatment versus 'passive' treatment was not defined by curability versus non–curability, but was based on the patient's perception of the doctor's level of *desire* to help them. In close relationships, therefore, even relatively minor palliative treatment could have as much significance and emotional importance as potentially curative therapy. Conversely, in distant relationships, even the promise of potential cure from the treatment was dulled if the doctor was perceived to be disinterested and not genuinely concerned for the patient in the process of administering therapy.

Bi-Directional Care: completing the picture

Completing the Model of Bi-Directional Care requires the specific incorporation of the doctor's need to be cared for and the patient's need to care. It is these features of role reversal as discussed in Chapter 4 and in the first section of this chapter that lend the model its name and represent the feature that distinguishes it most from other models (see Figure 5.4).

Role reversal within the Model of Bi-Directional Care did not necessarily threaten the stability or the validity of the doctor or the patient role. Rather, it merely saw their scope or definition widen as each became intermingled with elements of the other, particularly as distance between doctor and patient narrowed over time (see Figure 5.5).

The central axis of the Model of Bi-Directional Care is therefore a continuing care that is not rigidly *directional*. That is, continuing care did not only emanate *from* the doctor but also *to* the doctor, and was not only *received* by the patient but also *given* by them. Patient care for the doctor most often took the form of emotional or practical support (such as not calling the doctor after hours, the offering of tea and biscuits, or not offering any complaint if the doctor was running behind schedule).

FIGURE 5.4 The Model of Bi-Directional Care

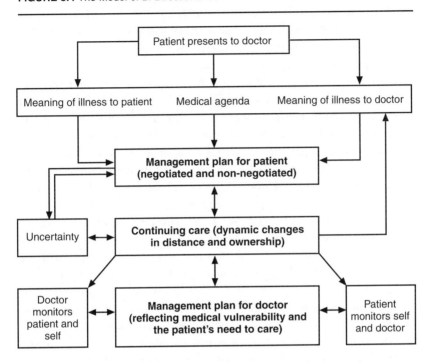

FIGURE 5.5 Links between doctor–patient distance and role reversal over time

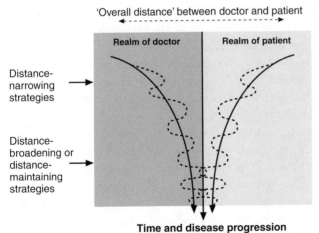

Time and disease progression
Progressive role ambiguity, role blurring and role reversal,
without obliterating the presence of the original role

Note: dotted lines represent fluctuation around the general trend, shown as unbroken lines

However, Chapter 4 also showed that patients and their families were capable of supporting the doctor in *medical* tasks. That was because their intimate familiarity with the illness made patients and their families quickly realise which medical interventions worked best for them. Sometimes, patients also had technically to *direct* the doctor in the execution of medical procedures in order to optimise their effectiveness.

The management plan for the doctor was an integral component of care that generally became more *pronounced* and more *necessary* as the continuity of care wore on. It became more pronounced as distance between doctor and patient narrowed and rapport between them strengthened (see Figure 5.5). Often, this related primarily to the patient's growing sensitivity for the doctor's needs and the patient's desire to offer such care, rather than to the necessity of such care. While the doctor's emotional anguish and need for care generally grew as the illness progressed, the outward manifestations of such a need remained highly variable. Sometimes it was openly manifest and definable, as in situations where their emotional anguish could not be hidden from patient and family. More often, however, the GP's need for care was more implicit rather than being verbally defined or visibly apparent. It was quietly manifest, based usually upon a combination of silent observations of the doctor's demeanour, as well as inferences about how the doctor must be feeling. The influence of this phenomenon, as indicated by the direction of the arrows in Figure 5.4, reverberated across all other facets of the process of care.

The above notion is virtually foreign to general practice literature, which generally sees continuity of care as rigidly unidirectional despite the fact that it well recognises medicine's shortcomings and its emotional challenges. McAvoy (1992: 81), for instance, emphasises unidirectional care when stating that 'while the doctor learns much about his [sic] patient over the years, the patient learns how much and what kind of help he [sic] can expect from his doctor'. Balint's (1964) notion of the person of the doctor as the therapeutic drug is also a far cry from the notion of the doctor *requiring* a therapeutic drug in the form of a caring patient.

Likewise, McWhinney (1989: 84, as quoted above on p. 171), in prohibiting the purpose of the doctor–patient relationship from being one which satisfies the doctor's 'own emotional needs', implies that the doctor–patient relationship is there for the *sole* benefit of the patient, not the doctor. The phenomenon of role reversal did not fully concur with this statement, because this statement suggests no scope for the doctor to validly and legitimately receive care from their patient in the context of a *proper relationship* whose prime purpose was to assist the patient. Role reversal showed that the doctor's own emotional needs (and sometimes even their very medical skills) could and did need to be supported. Further, such support was possible in a manner that was neither abusive to the nature of the doctor–patient relationship nor incompatible with the roles of doctor and patient. Rather, it in many ways enhanced the relationship by fully displaying medicine's human face and emotional responses to its very limitations, actions that facilitated the patient's need to actively care for their professional carers. Indeed, could this not be the ultimate expression of patient-centredness?

The palliative care literature, likewise, has not emphasised role reversal in any systematic way, even though it clearly recognises the manifold origins of emotional stress in doctors. Such understanding recognises the value of sharing uncertainty and anxiety with patients and families (although that was not always possible or appropriate, as Chapter 3 has demonstrated), but only in the context of such behaviour being professionally appropriate and compatible with a notion of keeping families informed about the illness. In this sense, the doctor is only secondarily cared for by patient and family, through the family's emotional preparation by the doctor for a potentially problematic illness course. Such a context of thinking does not emphasise enough the *active* nature of care that patient and family could offer the doctor (see also Chapter 3 on moral and emotional uncertainty), instead seeing professional colleagues or the doctor's own family and friends as more valid sources of care for them.

Chapter 4 showed that role reversal in close doctor–patient relationships could occur naturally and often subconsciously without threatening the social distinction between the doctor and the patient role. This suggested that such a tendency was *inherent* to those roles, even though its external manifestations were not always apparent. This tendency, however, had its limitations. The struggle, for example, to maintain an optimal distance represented attempts to safeguard the process of role reversal from becoming dysfunctional (that is, from reaching a point where an imbalance between caring versus receiving care transgressed social boundaries of acceptability in relation to one's role). Figure 5.5 diagrammatically summarises the dynamic links between doctor–patient distance and 'appropriate' or 'acceptable' role reversal over time. It is seen that over time, the close relationship was often concerned with distance-maintaining strategies rather than distance-narrowing strategies.

Conclusion: the significance of mutual care

The Model of Bi-Directional Care represents the culmination of this study of the nature and expression of medical power within the doctor–patient relationship. Rather than attempting to accurately describe all doctor–patient relationships, this model represents a particular kind of GP–cancer-patient relationship, one where doctor and patient have a close bond and mutual commitment to each other that resists the buffeting of clinical uncertainty and progressive illness. The preceding chapters have amply shown, however, that its derivation is centred as much upon the analysis of 'failed' or 'suboptimal' doctor–patient relationships as it is on 'successful' or 'good' relationships. Therefore, the Model of Bi-Directional Care has proven valuable in that the type of doctor–patient relationship that it describes has offered many new insights into the nature of medical power and the doctor–patient relationship.

In its essence, the Model of Bi-Directional Care forms a critique of the prescriptive patient-centred method of McWhinney (1989) by demonstrating the coexistence of a patient role within the doctor and a healer role within the patient. It does this by refocusing attention to the presence and person of the doctor in palliative care, and the impact of this presence on the nature of the doctor–patient relationship. By directly affecting doctor–patient dynamics, the doctor's own needs, vulnerabilities and reactions to the illness hold major repercussions for how the process of care is executed and experienced. This, in turn, opens up an active consideration of the patient as a valid and important giver of care *to* the doctor, in a process that does not destabilise the nature of the relationship but, on the contrary, strengthens it. The ultimate message is that the patient can no longer be understood in isolation from the doctor, just as the doctor cannot be understood in isolation from the patient.

In order to be properly contextualised, therefore, 'illness' and its 'healing' (as defined by Kleinman, 1978) have to incorporate these intricacies harboured within the doctor–patient relationship, particularly the 'fluidity' in doctor and patient roles. Such fluidity is located within the acceptable boundaries of the socially sanctioned roles of doctor and patient, and demonstrates that medical power, at its ultimate form of personalisation, is openly vulnerable. It is such 'controlled' vulnerability, however, that offers the patient new emotional opportunities (in terms of offering care to others) in situations where medical science itself has long been rendered powerless.

Indeed, depending upon the individual circumstances, the doctor's yielding to the care offered by the patient might in itself express the ultimate manifestation of true patient-centredness. Here, in the deepest personal recesses of the encounter between doctor and dying patient, the notion of medical power itself begins to break down and lose all relevance, becoming totally subsumed within the personal nature of their relationship.

Conclusion

The key challenge facing modern medicine is the humane and sensitive application of its scientific principles. The clinical encounter, unlike the laboratory experiment, is a *social* event that has had to rediscover what had been obscured by scientific rationalism—the principles of respect, caring and warmth. The patient-centred approach has contributed much in this quest, representing the pinnacle of efforts to rediscover the social presence of the patient. By actively integrating the patient's desires and feelings into the management plan, it set new standards for the clinical method.

However, the Model of Bi-Directional Care has evolved a step beyond the important advances made by the patient-centred approach, lending new insight into the nature of medical authority and practice. It has shown that the focus for patient-centredness (a 'movement' that has also gathered considerable political and medico-legal impetus) has diverted attention away from the person of the doctor and their own experience of illness.

A strongly role-bound notion of 'doctor' views the medical practitioner as emotionally and functionally neutral. Quite the contrary, however, has been demonstrated in this work. Doctors were vulnerable and had need of care, which patients themselves actively provided. This care helped to bolster the patients' own sense of self and self-esteem. Further, these processes did not threaten the stability of the doctor and patient roles, provided that the sense of ownership between doctor and patient was not excessive. This was the essence of bi-directional care. In short, the emotional responses, the needs and the *person* of the doctor *directly* influenced the nature of continuing care and indeed the very meaning and expression of patient-centredness itself. A phenomenology of the patient was so intimately intertwined with a phenomenology of the doctor that they could not be separated without the intricate dynamics of their relationship losing meaning and context.

The implications of these points for the understanding of medical power, the doctor–patient relationship, and the process of medical care have been significant. Medical authority, while strong, was simultaneously seen to be quite fragile and vulnerable. But it was precisely in its fragility that it gained additional strength. A medical authority that was *personalised*, transparently demonstrating its potential vulnerability, could resist the buffeting of progressive cancer illness and the universal presence of diverse forms of clinical uncertainty—factors that might otherwise confound and unsettle the strength of the doctor–patient relationship. Indeed, not only could the doctor–patient relationship resist decay under such influences, but was paradoxically capable of growing more *secure* as a result of them.

Public health policy and health planning have much to consider from these conclusions. The 'paradoxical' situation of burgeoning medico-legal action against doctors in this enlightened era of patient-centredness provides ample and urgent witness to such a statement. Public health policy needs to place a greater emphasis and value upon the stability and nature of the doctor–patient relationship, and its importance to the success of health interventions and outcomes. Health economics is also provided with a new dimension for consideration. The Model of Bi-Directional Care lends important perspective to the complex *human* nature of clinical interaction. It therefore also highlights the difficulty of incorporating such complexity into the costing of 'efficient' clinical practice using mathematical models alone.

The statements and conclusions so far drawn do *not* assume that the Model of Bi-Directional Care is set in 'theoretical concrete'. Derived from the setting of cancer care in general practice, the nature of the model and its more generalised applicability to wider spheres of medical practice could be subjected to further study. In particular, the nature of medical authority and the doctor–patient relationship could be examined in: (i) settings apart from general practice, (ii) in illness contexts apart from cancer, and (iii) in cultural contexts apart from Anglo-Australian and Greek-Australian.

The relationship between cancer patients and *specialist* doctors (such as oncologists, surgeons, intensive care physicians, psychiatrists and radiotherapists) might provide important comparisons and contrasts to the present observations of the GP–cancer patient relationship. How close, for example, is the specialist–cancer patient bond? Do specialists need to be cared for as actively as do GPs? How do they respond to efforts of patients to care for them? What is the nature of the care they receive? Are patients inclined to care for them as much as they are the GP? Furthermore, how does the specialist's relationship with their wider circle of peers and with the GP contribute to or affect such issues? The potential contrasts between adult cancer medicine and paediatric cancer medicine also provide scope for additional research. How applicable, for example, is 'bi-directionality' of care in the paediatric situation? If bi-directional care is applicable in this setting, what is its nature and quality?

Further from the field of cancer, the Model of Bi-Directional Care could also be tested in other medical settings of varying nature and duration, to see how it would be affected and to determine its applicability. In this context, chronic illness settings, such as those of osteoarthritis, congestive cardiac failure, chronic obstructive airways disease, diabetes mellitus or psychiatric illness, would provide valuable comparative study. Does serious illness that is not as directly life-threatening as cancer induce the same need within the doctor to be cared for, and within the patient to care for the doctor and for others around them? The same questions must also be asked in situations of relatively minor, self-limiting illness settings, such as common colds, influenza, acute bronchitis or gastroenteritis. Do these temporally restricted, (usually) non-threatening situations induce any sense of bi-directional care between doctor and patient and, if so, what is its nature and upon what does it depend?

Because the Model of Bi-Directional Care has been largely derived from accounts provided by Anglo-Australian (Anglo-Celtic) and Greek-Australian informants, an additionally important question relates to its degree of ethno-specificity. Although ethnicity was shown to influence how cancer illness and medical care were experienced, the Model of Bi-Directional Care makes no specific reference to it—it does not rely upon ethnicity as a distinct variable. The reason for this lay in the *similarities* of the illness experiences of the informants. *All*, for example, felt the threat of cancer, the need for hope, the struggle against uncertainty (particularly existential uncertainty), the need to be cared for and the need to actively reciprocate such care. These similarities suggested that such experiences, at their core, transcended ethnic boundaries, and instead evoked emotions and feelings that were more inherently founded upon human nature itself. However, the hypothetical extension of this observation to other cross-cultural contexts, while strongly plausible and inferred, is not certain. The nature and generalisability of the Model of Bi-Directional Care is therefore open to additional study across a wider variety of ethnic groups.

Future research agendas may wish to apply the Model of Bi-Directional Care to other forms of professional relationship outside the medical sphere. This would test both the applicability and the scope of the model, as well as potentially enhancing the existing understanding of such relationships. Examples of situations that are expected to harbour mutual caring might include the trading relationship between a retailer and a consumer, the academic relationship between a teacher and their pupil, the working relationship between an employer and their employee, or the political relationship between a Member of Parliament and one of their local constituents.

The potential relevance of the Model of Bi-Directional Care beyond the field of medicine ultimately relates to the fact that it probes an aspect common to all interpersonal relationships—an aspect that transcends the professional 'component' of those relationships. This aspect is the very humanity inherent in the interaction itself, which drives the process of mutual care.

Appendix

Implementation of the study framework

The research for this book was conducted through the University of Melbourne and approved by its Ethics Committee. All names appearing in this work are pseudonyms. The key elements of the study are as follows:

In-depth interviews

Individual, semi-structured in-depth interviews (Minichiello et al., 1990) with cancer patients who were living at home, their family carers, and general practitioners (GPs) were conducted. A family carer was defined as a person closely involved in the care of the patient. Patients and families were simply asked to talk about their experience of cancer illness and their interaction with the health system. GPs were asked to speak about their experiences in providing palliative care.

The interviews were audio-tape recorded in their entirety, and required the prior signing of an informed consent sheet. They were conducted in the major language of each informant, either English or Greek. All interviews were transcribed in full in preparation for analysis (Greek interviews were then translated into English). All interviews with doctors were in English.

Access to informants

Access to most patients and carers was via three Melbourne hospices that provided home-based palliative care: the Melbourne City Mission Hospice, the Southport Hospice and the Mercy Hospice. Patient and carer were interviewed in their home, usually separately. The identification of the carer was left to the family, and often the carer was a spouse. The end of the interview signalled the end of contact with the family. This basic protocol was also followed in recruiting several families directly through general practice—families that were not connected to the hospice system.

Access to GPs was via mail request. They were interviewed in their surgeries, either before or after clinical sessions. As with participating families, the end of the interview signalled the end of contact with the informant.

Sampling

Apart from cultural background, variety in the patient and carer informants was sought according to age, gender, English language proficiency, and type and duration of cancer illness. GP sampling likewise sought variety according to age, gender, practice type and location, and clinical experience. All GP informants were in active general practice. With the exception of one GP who looked after three of the participating families, the GP informants were not directly involved in caring for the patient and carer informants.

Analysis

Data from twelve families and ten GPs was obtained (Tables A.1 & A.2). The number of formal interviews completed is shown in Table A.3. Data was analysed at the individual level of the illness narrative (Good, 1994), and across individual stories according to the analytic induction method (Minichiello et al., 1990).

TABLE A.1 Summary of family informants

PARTICIPATING FAMILY	CONTACT LEVEL
[Maria, age 69 with breast cancer; Peter, age 74—husband; Greek]	Both formally interviewed
[Aristotle, age 79 with prostate cancer; Paula, age ?—daughter; Greek]	Aristotle too ill for interview; Paula formally interviewed
[George, age mid-50s with lung cancer; Katerina, age ?—wife; Greek]	Telephone contact only—George died before interview could be conducted.
[Paraskevi, age 48 with cervical cancer; Mark, age 23—son; Greek]	Introductory visit and detailed conversation but not formal interview
[Clare, age 65 with stomach cancer; Michael, age 67—husband; Anglo-Celtic]	Clare too ill for formal interview; Michael formally interviewed
[Charles, age 72 with prostate cancer; Amanda, age 72—wife; Anglo-Celtic]	Both formally interviewed
[Monica, age 48 with breast cancer; Alan, age late 50s—husband; Anglo-Celtic]	Both formally interviewed
[Barbara, age 48 with cervical cancer; Dimitri, age 53—husband; Greek]	Both formally interviewed
[Panteleimon, age 62 with lung cancer; Mary, age 63—wife; Greek]	Both formally interviewed
[Jane, English, age 61 with mycosis fungoides; John, German, age 70—husband]	Both formally interviewed
[Simon, age 64 with lymphoma; Cynthia, age 52—wife; Anglo-Celtic]	Both formally interviewed
[Brendan, age mid-40s with cerebral glioma; Michelle, age ?—wife; Anglo-Celtic]	Telephone contact only—Brendan did not feel up to a formal interview.

TABLE A.2 Summary of General Practitioner informants

[Carol, GP, age mid-30s; Anglo-Celtic]
[Frank, GP, age early 30s; Anglo-Celtic]
[Elizabeth, GP, age 32; Croatian]
[Byron, GP, age 57; Anglo-Celtic]
[Margarita, GP, age 33; Greek]
[Theodore, GP, age 63; Greek]
[Andrew, GP, age early 40s; Greek]
[Matthew, GP, age mid-30s; Greek]
[Anastasia, GP, age 31; Greek]
[Ben, GP, age 49; Jewish]

TABLE A.3 Informants who completed formal interviews

	PATIENTS	**CARERS**	**GPS**
Male	1 Greek	2 Greek	3 Greek
	2 Australian	2 Australian	2 Australian
			1 Jewish
Female	2 Greek	2 Greek	2 Greek
	1 Australian	2 Australian	1 Australian
	1 English		1 Croatian
Total	7	8	10
Age range	45–73 years	50–73 years	32–63 years

Bibliography

Adamson C. Existential and clinical uncertainty in the medical encounter: an idiographic account of an illness trajectory defined by inflammatory bowel disease and avascular necrosis. Sociology of Health and Illness 1997; 19(2): 133–159.

Ajzen I. Attitudes, Personality and Behaviour. Open University Press, Milton Keynes, 1988.

Aldridge D. Families, cancer and dying. Family Practice 1987 September; 4(3): 212–218.

Atkinson P. Training for certainty. Social Science and Medicine 1984; 19(9): 949–956.

Australian Institute of Health and Welfare. Australia's Health, 1996. The Fifth Biennial Report of the Australian Institute of Health and Welfare. Australian Government Publishing Service, Canberra, 1996.

Balint M. The Doctor, His Patient and the Illness. Second edition. Churchill Livingstone, Edinburgh, 1964 (reprinted 1986).

Becker G, Nachtigall RD. Ambiguous responsibility in the doctor–patient relationship: the case of infertility. Social Science and Medicine 1991; 32(8): 875–885.

Becker MH. Chapter 13: Psychosocial aspects of health-related behaviour (pp. 253–274), in Freeman HE, Levine S, Reeder LG (editors). Handbook of Medical Sociology. Third edition. Prentice-Hall Inc, Englewood Cliffs, New Jersey, 1979.

Bellamy M. GPs easy prey for violent patients. Australian Doctor (a weekly publication of Reed Business Information Pty Ltd, West Chatswood, New South Wales, Australia), 5 April, 1996, p. 58.

Berman HJ. The validity of role reversal: A hermeneutic perspective. Journal of Gerontological Social Work 1993; 20(3–4): 101–111.

Bloom SW, Wilson RN. Chapter 14: Patient–Practitioner Relationships (pp. 275–296), in Freeman HE, Levine S, Reeder LG (editors). Handbook of Medical Sociology. Third edition. Prentice-Hall Inc, Englewood Cliffs, New Jersey, 1979.

Bosk CL. Forgive and Remember. Managing Medical Failure. The University of Chicago Press, Chicago and London, 1979.

Brody EM. Role reversal: An inaccurate and destructive concept. Journal of Gerontological Social Work 1990; 15(1–2): 15–22.

Browne K, Freeling P. The Doctor–Patient Relationship. Second edition. Churchill Livingstone, Edinburgh, 1976.

Calnan M. Clinical uncertainty: is it a problem in the doctor–patient relationship? Sociology of Health and Illness 1984; 6(1): 74–85.

Cannon S. Social research in stressful settings: difficulties for the sociologist studying the treatment of breast cancer. Sociology of Health and Illness 1989; 11(1): 62–77.

Charlton RC. Attitudes towards care of the dying: a questionnaire survey of general practice attenders. Family Practice 1991 Dec; 8(4): 356–359.

Charmaz K. Loss of self: a fundamental form of suffering in the chronically ill. Sociology of Health and Illness 1983; 5(2): 168–195.

Charmaz K. 'Discovering' chronic illness using grounded theory. Social Science and Medicine 1990; 30(11): 1161–1172.

Craddock D. A Short Textbook of General Practice. Third edition. HK Lewis & Co, London, 1976.

Delvecchio-Good MJ. Discourses on Physician Competence (pp. 247–267), in: Hahn RA, Gaines AD (editors). Physicians of Western Medicine. D. Reidel Publishing Company, Dordrecht, 1985.

Delvecchio-Good MJ, Good BJ, Schaffer C, Lind SE. American oncology and the discourse on hope. Culture, Medicine and Psychiatry 1990 March; 14(1): 59–79.

Dickinson J, Lalor E, Calcino G, Douglass J, Knight R. Chapter 2: The Supply and Distribution of General Practitioners (pp. 25–64), in: Commonwealth Department of Health and Community Services. General Practice in Australia. Australian Government Publishing Service, Canberra, 1996.

Dozor RB, Addison RB. Toward a good death: an interpretive investigation of family practice residents' practices with dying patients. Family Medicine 1992 Sept–Oct; 24(7): 538–543.

Engel G. The need for a new medical model: A challenge for biomedicine. Science 1977; 196: 129–136.

Ferguson B, Browne E (editors). Health Care and Immigrants. A Guide for the Health Professionals. MacLennan & Petty Pty Ltd, Sydney, 1991.

Fisher S. Doctor–patient communication: a social and micropolitical performance. Sociology of Health and Illness 1984; 6(1): 1–29.

Foucault M. The Birth of the Clinic. An Archaeology of Medical Perception. (Translated from the French by A.M. Sheridan Smith). Vintage Books. A Division of Random House Inc, New York, 1994.

Fox R. Training for Uncertainty (pp. 207–241), in: Merton RK, Reader G, Kendall P (editors). The Student-Physician. Harvard University Press, Cambridge, 1957.

Fraser RC (editor). Clinical Method. A General Practice Approach. Second edition. Butterworth-Heinemann Ltd, Oxford, 1992.

Freeman WL, Altice P, Betton HB, Lincoln JA, Robbins CM. Care of the dying patient. The Journal of Family Practice 1976 Oct; 3(5): 547–555.

Gelder M, Gath D, Mayou R. Oxford Textbook of Psychiatry. Oxford University Press, Oxford, 1986.

Glaser B, Strauss A. Awareness of Dying. Aldine Publishing Company, Chicago, 1965.

Glaser B, Strauss A. Status Passage. Routledge & Kegan Paul, London, 1971.

Good BJ. Medicine, Rationality and Experience. An Anthropological Perspective. Cambridge University Press, Cambridge, 1994.

Gordon DR. Embodying illness, embodying cancer. Culture, Medicine and Psychiatry 1990 June; 14(2): 275–297.

Groopman LC. Medical internship as moral education: An essay on the system of training physicians. Culture, Medicine and Psychiatry 1987; 11: 207–227.

Helman CG. Culture, Health and Illness. An Introduction for Health Professionals. Second edition. Butterworth Heinemann, Oxford, 1990.

Hetzel B. Health and Australian Society. Third edition. Penguin Books, Victoria, Australia, 1982.

Hugo G, Maher C. Atlas of the Australian People—1991 Census (National Overview). Australian Government Publishing Service, Canberra, 1995.

Hull R. A Pocketbook of Palliative Care. McGraw Hill, Sydney, 1994.

Jewson ND. The disappearance of the sick man from medical cosmology, 1770–1870. Sociology 1976; 10(2): 225–244.

Kamien M. Academic general practice comes of age? Australian Family Physician 1997; 26 (Suppl 1): S47–S49.

Katz P. How Surgeons Make Decisions (pp. 155–175), in: Hahn RA, Gaines AD (editors). Physicians of Western Medicine. D. Reidel Publishing Company, Dordrecht, 1985.

Kellehear A. Are we a death denying society? A sociological review. Social Science and Medicine 1984; 18(9): 713–723.

Kellehear A. Dying of Cancer. The Final Year of Life. Harwood Academic Publishers, London, 1990.

Kellehear A. Chapter 12: The Social Inequality of Dying (pp. 181–189), in: Waddell C, Petersen AR (editors). Just Health. Inequality in Illness, Care and Prevention. Churchill Livingstone, Melbourne, 1994.

Kellehear A. Chapter 18: Health and the Dying Person (pp. 287–299), in: Waddell C, Petersen A (editors). Health Matters. Allen & Unwin, Sydney, 1998.

Kellehear A, Fook J. Chapter 34: Sociological Factors in Death Denial by the Terminally Ill (pp. 527–537), in: Sheppard JL (editor). Advances in Behavioural Medicine, Volume 6. Cumberland College of Health Sciences, Sydney, 1989.

Kleinman A. Clinical relevance of anthropological and cross-cultural research: concepts and strategies. American Journal of Psychiatry 1978 April; 135(4): 427–431.

Kubler-Ross E. On Death and Dying. MacMillan Publishing Co, Inc, New York, 1969.

Kumar P, Clark M (editors). Clinical Medicine. A Textbook for Medical Students and Doctors. Third edition. Bailliere Tindall, London, 1994.

Kune GA, Kune S, Watson LF. Perceived religiousness is protective for colorectal cancer: data from The Melbourne Colorectal Cancer Study. Journal of the Royal Society of Medicine 1993 Nov; 86: 645–647.

Light D. Uncertainty and control in professional training. Journal of Health and Social Behaviour 1979; 20: 310–322.

Lloyd GER (editor). Hippocratic Writings (translated by Chadwick J, Mann WN, Lonie IM, Withington ET). Penguin Books, London, 1983.

Lossky V. The Mystical Theology of the Eastern Church. St Vladimir's Seminary Press, Crestwood, New York, 1976.

MacLennan AH. Who will deliver the next generation? Medical Journal of Australia 1993 Aug; 159: 261–263.

Maseide P. Possibly abusive, often benign, and always necessary. On power and domination in medical practice. Sociology of Health and Illness 1991; 13(4): 545–561.

McAvoy PA. Chapter 5: The Doctor–Patient Relationship (pp. 78–92), in: Fraser RC (editor). Clinical Method. A General Practice Approach. Second edition. Butterworth-Heinemann Ltd, Oxford, 1992.

McCormick J. The Doctor. Father Figure or Plumber. Croom Helm, London, 1979.

McWhinney IR. A Textbook of Family Medicine. Oxford University Press, New York, 1989.

Mechanic D. Chapter 4: The Patient's Perspective of His Illness: The Study of Illness Behaviour (pp. 115–157); in Mechanic D. Medical Sociology. A Selective View. The Free Press, New York, 1968.

Minichiello V, Aroni R, Timewell E, Alexander L. In-depth Interviewing. Researching People. Longman Cheshire Pty Ltd, Melbourne, 1990.

Mitchell G. Nothing ventured, nothing gained. Medical Observer (a fortnightly publication of Medical Observer Pty Ltd, Seaforth, New South Wales, Australia), 19 September 1997, p. 7.

Miyaji N. The power of compassion: truth telling among American doctors in the care of dying patients. Social Science and Medicine 1993; 36(3): 249–264.

Morgan M. Chapter 4: The Doctor–Patient Relationship (pp. 46–64), in: Scambler G (editor). Sociology as Applied to Medicine. Third edition. Bailliere Tindall, London, 1991.

Morrell DC. An Introduction to Primary Medical Care. Churchill Livingstone, Edinburgh, 1976.

Murtagh J. General Practice. McGraw-Hill Book Company, Sydney, 1994.

Naish J, Brown J, Denton B. Intercultural consultations: Investigation of factors that deter non-English speaking women from attending their general practitioners for cervical screening. British Medical Journal 1994 Oct; 309: 1126–1128.

National Health Strategy. Removing Cultural and Language Barriers to Health. National Health Strategy Issues Paper No. 6, Treble Press, 1993 (Place of publication not listed in this Australian document).

O'Driscoll M. Chapter 12: Attitude Change (pp. 294–307), in: Gardner G, Innes JM, Forgas JP, O'Driscoll M, Pearce PL & Newton JW. Social Psychology. Prentice Hall of Australia, Sydney, 1981.

Parsons T. The Social System. Routledge & Kegan Paul Ltd, London, 1951.

Rosen G. The Hospital: Historical Sociology of a Community Institution (pp. 1–36), in: Freidson E (editor). The Hospital in Modern Society. The Free Press (A division of Macmillan Publishing Co. Inc), New York, 1963.

Rosser JE, Maguire P. Dilemmas in general practice: The care of the cancer patient. Social Science and Medicine 1982; 16: 315–322.

Saillant F. Discourse, knowledge and experience of cancer: a life story. Culture, Medicine and Psychiatry 1990 March; 14(1): 81–104.

Shorter E. Bedside Manners. The Troubled History of Doctors and Patients. Simon and Schuster, New York, 1985.

Siegler M. Searching for moral certainty in medicine: A proposal for a new model of the doctor–patient encounter. Bulletin of the New York Academy of Medicine 1981; 57: 56–69.

Silverman D. Communication and Medical Practice. Social Relations in the Clinic. Sage Publications, London, 1987.

Skolbekken JA. The risk epidemic in medical journals. Social Science and Medicine 1995; 40(3): 291–305.

Snyder M. 'Becoming': A method for expanding systemic thinking and deepening empathic accuracy. Family Process 1995 June; 34: 241–253.

Sontag S. Illness as Metaphor. Farrer, Starus & Giroux, New York, 1978.

Southern Sydney Area Health Service. Health for Multicultural Australia: National Agenda for Multicultural Health in Australia, May 1994. A Report on the Plenary Deliberations and Recommendations from the National Conference 'Health for Multicultural Australia' held at Sydney University, November 10–12, 1993. (pp. 13–16).

Stevens J. Talking shop. Australian Family Physician 1994 May; 23(5): 785.

Still AW, Todd CJ. Role ambiguity in general practice: the care of patients dying at home. Social Science and Medicine 1986; 23(5): 519–525.

Stimson G, Webb B. Going to See the Doctor. The Consultation Process in General Practice. Routledge & Kegan Paul, London, 1975.

Strauss A, Corbin J, Faberhaugh S, Glaser B, Maines D, Suczek B, Weiner CL. Chronic Illness and the Quality of Life. The CV Mosby Company, St Louis, 1984.

Strong PM. The Ceremonial Order of the Clinic. Patients, Doctors and Medical Bureaucracies. Routledge & Kegan Paul, London, 1979.

Strong PM. Viewpoint: the academic encirclement of medicine? Sociology of Health and Illness 1984; 6(3): 339–358.

Toulmin S. Cosmopolis. The Hidden Agenda of Modernity. The Free Press (A division of Macmillan, Inc), New York, 1990.

Twaddle AC. The concept of health status. Social Science and Medicine 1974; 8: 29–38.

Vafiadis P. The dilemma of the unexpected result. Australian Family Physician 1996 June; 25(6): 971, 973, 975.

Vanderwoude JC. Chapter 12: The Caregiver as Patient (pp. 119–126), in: Van Eys J & McGovern JP (editors). The Doctor as a Person. Charles C Thomas, Publisher, Springfield, Illinois, USA, 1988.

Waddington I. The role of the hospital in the development of modern medicine: A sociological analysis. Sociology 1973; 7(2): 211–224.

West C. Reconceptualising gender in physician–patient relationships. Social Science and Medicine 1993; 36 (1): 57–66.

Willis E. Medical Dominance. The Division of Labour in Australian Health
Care. George Allen & Unwin, Sydney, 1983.

Woodruff R. Palliative Medicine. Symptomatic and Supportive Care for Patients
with Advanced Cancer and AIDS. Asperula Pty Ltd, Melbourne, 1993.

Young A. The creation of medical knowledge: some problems in interpretation.
Social Science and Medicine 1981; 15B: 379–386.

Index

acupuncture, 81, 117
Adamson, C., 16, 115, 121
Addison, R. B., 39, 61,
 118, 156
adjustment, 85–7
Ajzen, I., 4
Ajzen's Theory of Planned
 Behaviour, 4, 5
Aldridge, D., 60, 155
Alexander, L., 21
alternative medicine, 15, 81,
 116, 117, 118
Altice, P., 111
Aroni, R., 21
Atkinson, P., 100, 103,
 121, 122
Australian Institute of
 Health and Welfare, 14
authority
 challenge to, 4
 of medical profession,
 3–4
awareness
 categories in terminal
 illness, 70
 closed, 70
 discounted, 65, 66, 70
 mutual-pretence, 70
 open, 70
 partial, 70
 suspected, 70, 74

Balint, M., 7, 11, 174
Becker, G., 111

Becker, M. H., 4
bedside medicine, 3
Bellamy, M., 12, 14
Berman, H. J., 150
Betton, H. B., 111
Bi-directional Care, Model
 of, 159, 167–77
bio-psycho-social approach,
 7, 10, 76
Bloom, S. W., 7
Bosk, C. L., 110, 112, 120,
 121, 122, 162
Brody, E. M., 145, 150
Brown, J., 134
Browne, E., 19
Browne, K., 168, 169

Calcino, G., 12
Calnan, M., 111, 121, 122
cancer
 as a determined
 outcome, 45–6
 as disease and non-self,
 25–6
 as gain, 32
 as interaction, 26–8
 as loss, 28
 naming, 68
 as self, 37–40
 as struggle, 35–7
 as taboo, 22–4
 as a test, 43–5
 as uncertain or
 unknown, 40–3

cancer world
 of GP, 46–61
 of patient and carer,
 22–46
Cannon, S., 142
care
 and the concept of
 direction in
 bi-directional, 167–75
 traditional concepts, 4–5
carer, 21
Charlton, R. C., 18
Charmez, K., 15, 21, 28,
 39, 86, 115
Chinese herb medicine,
 81, 117
chronicity emphasis,
 47, 56–8
Clark, M., 12, 47, 102
client, 15, 155
communication, 67, 107–10
 non-verbal, 85, 132
compatibility between
 doctor and patient see
 harmony between
 doctor and patient
complementary medicine,
 15, 37, 116
compliance, 4
 lack of, 82
compromise, 107
consultant see specialist
consumer, 15, 115
control, in the

doctor–patient
relationship, 6–7
Corbin, J., 86, 89, 90, 94
counter-transference,
145, 169
Craddock, D. A., 145, 169
cross-cultural experiences,
19–20
culture
compatibility in
doctor–patient
relationship,
108, 133–4
difference in acceptance
of cancer, 22
disclosure, different
attitudes, 73
education differences, 42
effect on doctor–patient
relationship, 59
gender specific issue, 89
language, 134
non-disclosure, 84
opinions of general
practitioners,
130, 131
social distance, 132–3
cupping, 81, 117
curing, 8, 157
versus healing, 8

death, 23
defensive medicine, 14
Delvecchio-Good, M. J.,
37, 40, 110, 113
Denton, B., 134
dermatologist, 38
diagnosis
models of diagnostic
delay, 109
second diagnosis, 69
Dickinson, J., 12
disclosure
awareness in, 69–70
direction and sequence
in, 72–3
dynamics of, 72–4
emotive and non-verbal
content of, 75
gradual, 66
key conclusions about,
75–6
multiplicity in, 74
nature and purpose, 69
non-verbal, 66
pre-disclosure, 67–8

source of, 72
timing of, 70, 74
verbal, 66
disease
versus illness, 8, 157
disease-burden emphasis,
47, 50–2
distance
dependence on
ownership, 137
doctor-patient, 125
emotional, 135–7
optimal, 140–2
optimising, 140–4
ownership, role reversal
and medical power,
154–7
professional, 127–32
social, 132–5
value of, 142
doctor
morality, sense of, 135
new, 14–15
role, 6
stress, 111, 148
doctor–family interaction,
63–9
doctor–patient
communication, 67
distance between, 127
partnership, 47, 58–60
relationship, models of,
6–8
Douglass, J., 12
Dozer, R. B., 39, 61,
118, 156

Engel, G., 7, 76
environmental factors, 45–6
epidemiological emphasis,
47, 48–50
error, 15, 101, 121
ethics, 8, 13, 73, 102
relationship between
medical power and,
163–4
euthanasia, 8, 119, 120

Faberhaugh, S., 86, 89,
90, 94
Family Medicine
Movement, 8
fear, 29, 56
female doctors, 11–12,
112, 132
Ferguson, B., 19

Fisher, S., 103, 124
Fook, J., 15
Foucault, M., 3, 99
Fox, R., 13, 99, 100, 101,
103, 121
Fraser, R. C., 65
Freeling, P., 167, 169
Freeman, W. L., 111
friendship, 141
functional emphasis,
47, 52–4

Gath, D., 145, 150
Gelder, M., 145, 150
gender, 11–12
social distance, 132
general practice
opinion of, 8, 130, 131
setting, 18–19
general practitioners
coping, 75
effects of medical
uncertainty, 123
ethics, 73
falsifying information, 73
general practitioner views of
cancer
chronicity emphasis,
47, 56–8
disease-burden emphasis,
47, 50–2
epidemiological
emphasis, 47, 48–50
functional emphasis,
47, 52–4
intuitive emphasis,
47, 54–6
partnership emphasis,
47, 58–60
Glaser, B., 12, 63, 69, 81, 86,
89, 90, 94, 111, 152, 164
God, 43, 145
Good, B. J., 5, 8, 18, 37,
40, 62, 68
Gordon, D. R., 37, 76
Groopman, L. C., 49,
119, 162

habit-related factors, 45
harmony between doctor
and patient
cultural and language
issues in, 107–10
impact on uncertainty,
96–7
prerequisites for, 93–6

threat posed by uncertainty, 98
healing, 8
Health Belief Model, 4, 65
health promotion, 4, 37
Helman, C. G., 12, 19
Hetzel, B., 14
Hippocratic
  Oath, 2
  writings, 2
home, 87–90
home-based care
  benefits, 87–8
  inherent risks in, 88–9
  remedies, 65, 80
  social distance,
    narrowing, 134
hope, 30, 51, 55
hospital, 87–90
  medicine, 3
Hugo, G., 20
Hull, R. A., 54, 76, 118

identity
  of doctor, 17
  hierarchies, 115
  of patient, 17, 86
  preferred, 86, 115
Illness Behaviour Model,
  4, 5
illness
  progression, 64
  versus disease, 8
informed consent, 9
intuitive emphasis, 47, 54–6
investigations see tests

Jewson, N. D., 2, 3

Kamien, M., 8
Katz, P., 103, 110
Kellehear, A., 3, 15, 18, 41,
  69, 70, 72, 86, 113, 135
Kleinman, A., 8, 157, 176
Knight, R., 12
Kubler-Ross, E., 50, 86
Kumar, P., 12, 47, 102
Kune, G. A., 11
Kune, S., 11

laboratory medicine, 3
Lalor, E., 12
language
  limitations in, 107–10
  primary importance over
    culture in

doctor–patient
  interactions, 134
Light, D., 101, 103, 106,
  107, 108, 121
Lincoln, J. A., 111
Lind, S. E., 37, 40
litigation, 13, 15, 17, 91
Lloyd, G. E. R., 2
loss, 29, 31, 39
  minimisation of, 29–30
Lossky, V., 145, 150

MacLennan, A. H., 13
Maguire, P., 10, 19, 103
Maher, C., 20
Maines, D., 86, 89, 90, 94
malpractice, 15
mammography, 68
Maseide, P., 10, 16, 98, 138
Mayou, R., 145, 150
McAvoy, P. A., 145, 169, 174
McCormick, J., 145, 169
McWhinney, I. R., 9, 12,
  145, 157, 167, 169, 171,
  174, 176
meaning-centred tradition, 8
Mechanic, D., 4
medical advances, 3, 13
medical authority see
  medical power
medical hierarchy, 107,
  110, 129
medical power
  actual versus perceived,
    17
  distance, ownership and
    role reversal,
    implication for,
    154–7
  expression, 93
  form, 90–1, 161–2
  key questions in, 8–9, 90
  location, 91–3
  nature and quality of, 93
  patient-centred
    approach, 156–7
  relationship between
    ethics and, 163–4
  summary of, 159–66
medical profession
  collective power, 91
  uncertainty in,
    100–2, 121–2
medico-legal liability, 113
mental faculties, loss of, 29
Minichiello, V., 21

minimisation of loss, 39
Mitchell, G., 104
Miyaji, N., 70, 76
Model of Bi-Directional
  Care, 159, 167–77
Model of Illness Behaviour,
  4, 5
models of the
  doctor–patient
    relationship, 6–8
monitoring
  according to response
    and progress, 84
  actions and reactions of
    others, 85
  appearance, 83
  by comparison, 84–5
  functional, 82
  the treatment type, 83
  via investigations, 83–4
moral issues see ethics
Morrell, D. C., 167
multidisciplinary care,
  disadvantages of, 76, 11
multidisciplinary team,
  60, 110
Murtagh, J., 168

Nachtigall, R. D., 111
Naish, J., 134
naming the illness, 68
National Health Strategy, 19
negotiation, 169
'new' doctor, 11–14
'new' patient, 14–15
'New Public Health'
  movement, 4
non-disclosure, 84
  to family, 28
  patient protecting, 69
non-Hodgkin's lymphoma,
  68
non-verbal communication,
  85
normalisation, 31, 50

O'Driscoll, M., 145
oncologist, 37, 79, 101
ownership
  dependence on distance,
    137–42, 154–7
  excessive, 142–4

palliative care, 18, 52–3
Papanicolaou smear test,
  37, 68

Parsons, T., 6
partnership emphasis,
47, 58–60
patient, 15
'new', 14–15
role, 6
patient-centred approach, 16
medical power, 156–7
Patient-Centred Clinical
Method, 9
evolution, 8–10
limitations, 10–11
strengths, 9–10
physician, 2
power, 90–3, 98
pre-disclosures, 67–8
preventive medicine, 4
psycho-neuro-immunology,
118
qualitative method, 5

relationship see
doctor–patient
relationship
religion, 33, 43–4, 118, 119,
124, 134, 145
responsibility, 110–12
risk, 92, 104
calculation, 13
epidemic, 11
risk-taking, 92
Robbins, C. M., 111
role
of doctor, 6
of patient, 6
role-distancing, 15
role-forcing, 12, 94, 111
role-reversal
description, 146–9
distance, ownership and
medical power,
154–7
introduction to, 144–5
properties of, 149–54
Rosen, G., 2, 3
Rosser, J. E., 10, 19, 103, 106

Saillant, F., 40, 76
Schaffer, C., 37, 40
scientific method, 3–4
second cancer diagnosis, 69
self, 44
loss of, 15
self-control, 44
Shorter, E., 15
Siegler, M., 120, 157

Silverman, D., 9, 10, 16,
98, 138
Skolbekken, J. A., 11, 13
Snyder, M., 151
Sontag, S., 22, 23, 25, 32,
37, 40
Southern Sydney Area
Health Service, 109,
133, 134
specialisation, 8
specialist, 59, 100
effects of medical
uncertainty on,
121–2
Stevens, J., 145
Still, A. W., 106, 156, 161
Stimson, G., 127, 132,
136, 167
Strauss, A., 12, 63, 69, 82, 86,
89, 90, 94, 111, 153, 164
stress, 37, 89
in doctors, 148
Strong, P. M., 110, 136
sub-specialisation, 8
Suczek, B., 86, 89, 90, 94

technology, 3, 13
impact on
doctor–patient
relationship, 95
tests, 83, 95, 114
threats of illness to doctor,
23
Timewell, E., 21
Todd, C. J., 106, 156, 161
total care, 18
Toulmin, S., 2, 5, 11
transference, 145
treatment
active. versus passive,
76–80
alternative, 15
complexity and
invasiveness, 78
medical, 77, 79
non-medical, 80–1
passive, 7
prolonging life versus
hastening death,
96–7, 119
rapidity, 78–9
synchronising to patient
expectations, 81–2
trust, 58, 59, 74, 77
truth
balancing, 49–50

difficulty in defining,
70–1
falsification of, 73
importance, 69
patient protecting, 41
Twaddle, A. C., 65

uncertainty
as a clinical tool, 76
effects of, on
bi-directional care,
170–2
existential, 115–16
future, patient, 29
inherent, 113, 116
inter-personal, 106–7
knowledge-related, 99
in locating responsibility,
110
moral and emotional,
118–20
need to be viewed
concurrently with
certainty, 121–2
in negotiating different
illness paradigms,
116–18
process-related,
105–6, 113
as a reflection of
doctor–patient
compatibility, 122–4
related to health-care
structure, 103, 105
technical, 112–13

Vafiadis, P., 13, 67, 83
Vanderwoude, J. C., 10, 150
vulnerability
of doctor, 88
of patient, 176

Waddington, I., 3
Watson, L. F., 11
Webb, B., 127, 132, 136, 167
Weiner, C. L., 86, 89, 90, 94
West, C., 12
whole-patient approach, 78
Willis, E., 9, 11, 145
Wilson, R. N., 7
Woodruff, R., 18
work factors, 45–5

Young, A., 103